推拿手法图解

汉英对照 Chinese-English Edition

沈国权 严隽陶 编著
WRITTEN BY SHEN GUOQUAN AND YAN JUNTAO

李承建 绘图
DRAWN BY LI CHENGJIAN

Illustrations Of Tuina Manipulations

上海科学技术出版社
SHANGHAI SCIENTIFIC & TECHNICAL PUBLISHERS

图书在版编目(CIP)数据

推拿手法图解(汉英对照)/沈国权,严隽陶编著.—上海:上海科学技术出版社,2004.1
ISBN 7-5323-7120-4

Ⅰ.汉... Ⅱ.①沈...②严... Ⅲ.推拿疗法(中医)
—图解 Ⅳ.R244.1-64

中国版本图书馆 CIP 数据核字(2003)第 047362 号

上海科学技术出版社出版、发行
(上海瑞金二路450号 邮政编码200020)
苏州望电印刷有限公司印刷
新华书店上海发行所经销
2004年1月第1版 2004年1月第1次印刷
开本 787×1092 1/16 印张 11.5 字数 190 千
印数 1—4 200
定价：35.00元

本书如有缺页、错装或坏损等严重质量问题，
请向本社出版科联系调换

内容提要

Content Summary

本书是一本用中英文对照编写的推拿手法图解，全书共分 3 章。第一章概论，介绍了推拿手法的分类、作用途径及技术要求；第二章推拿手法，详细地介绍了按压类手法、推擦类手法、摩揉类手法等 14 类手法；第三章推拿操作常规，介绍了头面部、颈项部、肩部等身体 10 个部位的操作规则。

本书内容丰富，绘图准确，每图均抓住推拿手法的动作要领，勾划出掌握推拿手法操作的切入点，不仅对推拿手法的初学者提供帮助，而且对推拿科的临床医师进一步发挥手法的治疗作用也颇有裨益。

This is an atlas of Tuina manipulations written in collated Chinese with English. The book is divided in 3 chapters. The manipulation classification, mechanism approach and technical requirements are introduced in the first chapter. In the second chapter, manipulations of 14 categories such as the pressing category, the linear-moving category, the circular-moving category etc. are described. And all the routine techniques on different body parts such as on the head and facial regions, the neck and nape regions, the shoulder region are also delineated in the last chapter.

With abundant manipulation resources and accurate drawings, this works is not an ecumenic iconography book of Tuina manipulation. Reversal, the authors focalize at the motion conspectus of the manipulations to depict out of the incision

Content Summary

point, at which you will be easy to control skills of all manipulations. Thus it is not only helpful for the beginner to learn Tuina manipulation, but beneficial for the clinician to elevate the therapeutic effect of manipulation as well.

前言 Preface

推拿是人类最早掌握的医疗方法之一。经过数千年的曲折发展之后,这一古老的疗法又被人类重新认识,焕发出新的青春活力。人们深信,作为一种无痛、无毒副反应、非损伤性、不介入人体的自然疗法,推拿必将在人类的卫生保健事业中发挥更大的作用。

推拿手法是推拿治疗的基本手段。由于推拿手法本身是一种富于技巧的人体运动形式,很难以文字精确地加以描述,学习手法者也难以仅凭文字描述正确地理解手法操作方式及将此手法操作正确地表现还原。南辕北辙,以非为是者,大有人在。

作者从多年的教学工作中体会到,形象教学在推拿手法教学中远比理论教学更为重要。一幅简单的图片所包含的信息量远远超过一篇数百字的文章。故决定编撰推拿手法图解,以飨读者。

本书收录了中外推拿手法近200种,是迄今同类书籍中收集较为丰富的。其中的矫正性手法在本书中尤占有重要的地位,算是本书的特色吧!本书的编写以图为主,配以文字说明。对于一些操作较为复杂而临床较为常用的推拿手法,予以动态图描绘,以利读者理解掌握。为了不但让中国读者了解国内推拿手法,也让国外同行了解中国推拿手法,本书采用了中英文对照排版。对于初学推拿者来说,本书文字浅显,绘图精确,在阅读上不致有什么困难。对于推拿专业人员来说,本书的手法分类体系和对手法的演变分析及最新介绍的国外推拿手法,也将给他们带来裨益。

本书在1994年出版以后,蒙读者错爱,很快脱销,超出了作者和出版社的预料。此次借再版之际,对原书的错误进行了一些修正,

Preface

并向广大读者表示感谢。但因作者水平所限，其中的错误在所难免，望读者能予以进一步指正。

沈国权 严隽陶

2002 年 7 月

Tuina is one of the oldest therapies that human being has controlled. After tortuous development of thousands years, this old therapeutics freshes a new vigor again and is recognized by mankind. It is deeply believed that, as a natural therapeutics of no pain, no side effect, no poison, no injurious, and no interfere in body, Tuina will play a more important role in man's health enterprise.

Manipulation is the essential procedure of Tuina therapy. Since the manipulation is skillful and dexterous movement of the body, it is difficult to be described accurately in words. And for the learners, it is also difficult to understand and master the manipulative manner rightly by means of writing or manipulated correctly from reading books. There are a lot of persons who try to go south but drive car according north chariot and take wrong as right in studying Tuina manipulation.

From the practical work of dozens years, we have gotten the idea that diagrams are better than word descriptions in Tuina teaching. A piece of simplest diagram contains more information than an article of hundreds words does. So we decided to compile this book to satisfy readers.

Approximately two hundred Tuina manipulations originated

from both China and foreign countries are compiled in this book. Maybe it is one of abounds sorts of manipulation book so far. Moreover, the rectifying manipulations especially occupy an outstanding role in this book and thus make it distinguished from other Tuina books. We take the diagrams as main form and the word illustrations as supporting role in our complement work. Some manipulations that are difficulty learned and frequently used in clinic are drawn in series of diagrams, so that the reader will be easy to understand them. In order to that, let not only Chinese reader master Tuina manipulation, but the foreign reader understand manipulation of China as well, this book adapts the comparing typesetting of Chinese and English. For the beginners of Tuina, the writing of this book is plain and simple, and the drawn is meticulous. So they will have no difficult in reading. For the specialized persons, the classification system of manipulation, the evolution analysis of manipulation and the late introduction of foreign manipulations in this book will also bring them a lot of benefit.

Since the publishing of the first version in 1994, the book has received preference from the readers and has been sold out soon. It is beyond the anticipation of the writers and the publishers. Even though we have corrected some mistakes in the first version, there still are wrong in this book. We give expression of thankfulness to your readers. And we also hope you will set right for us.

Shen Guoquan Yan Juntao

July, 2002

目 录
CONTENTS

第一章 概论
CHAPTER 1 INTRODUCTION

第一节　手法的分类 4
SECTION 1 CLASSIFICATION OF THE MANIPULATIONS

第二节　推拿手法的作用途径 6
SECTION 2 EFFECTING PROCESSES OF THE MANIPULATIONS

第三节　推拿手法的技术要求 7
SECTION 3 TECHNICAL REQUIREMENTS OF TUINA MANIPULATIONS

1.刺激性手法的技术要求 7
1.Technical requirement of stimulating manipulations

2.矫正性、松动性手法的技术要求 8
2.Technical requirements of rectifying and mobilizing manipulations

第二章 推拿手法
CHAPTER 2 TUINA MANIPULATIONS

第一节　按压类手法 13
SECTION 1 CATEGORY OF PRESSING MANIPULATIONS

一、代表手法　按法 13
Principal Techniques of Pressing Manipulations: Pressing

1.指按法 14
1.Pressing with thumb

2.掌按法 14
2.Pressing with palm

目录 / Contents

二、按法的衍化 15
Evolution of Pressings
  1.肘压法 15
  1.Compressing with the elbow
  2.点法 16
  2.Pointing
  3.掐法 17
  3.Nipping with the thumbnail
  4.押法 18
  4.Touching
  5.掩法、扪法 18
  5.Cupping, Warm covering

三、按压复位法 18
Pressing-Reductions
  1.寰枕关节按压复位法 20
  1.Pressing-Reduction of the atlantooccipital joint
  2.上颈椎侧卧位按压复位法 21
  2.Pressing-reduction of the upper cervical vertebrae in laterallying position
  3.下颈椎俯卧位按压复位法 21
  3.Pressing-reduction of the lower cervical vertebrae in prone position
  4.上胸椎按压复位法 22
  4.Pressing-reduction of the upper thoracic vertebrae in prone position
  5.上胸椎指拨复位法 22
  5.Bending-reduction of the upper thoracic vertebrae with the thumb
  6.胸椎交叉按压复位法 23
  6.Cross pressing-reduction of the thoracic vertebrae
  7.胸椎棘突下掌缘按压复位法 23
  7.Pressing-reduction upon the spinous process of the thoracic vertebrae with palm rim
  8.肋椎关节按压复位法 24
  8.Pressing-reduction of the costovertebral joint
  9.骶髂关节按压松动法 24
  9.Pressing-mobilization of the sacroiliac joint

第二节 推擦类手法 25
SECTION 2 CATEGORY OF LINEAR-MOVING MANIPULATIONS

一、代表手法 推法 26
Principal Techniques of Linear-moving Manipulations: Pushing
  1.拇指直推法 26
  1.Linear-pushing with the thumb

2.剑指直推法 26
　　2.Linear-pushing with the "sword-fingers"
　　3.拇指平推法 27
　　3.Flat-pushing with the thumb
　　4.掌平推法 27
　　4.Flat-pushing with the palm
　　5.刨推法 28
　　5.Planing-pushing
　　6.拳平推法 28
　　6.Flat-pushing with the fist
　　7.肘平推法 29
　　7.Flat-pushing with the elbow
　　8.分推法与合推法 29
　　8.Eccentric-pushing and concentric-pushing

二、推法的衍化 30
　　Evolution of Pushing
　　1.擦法 30
　　1.Linear-rubbing
　　2.拨法 32
　　2.Plucking
　　3.抹法 32
　　3.Wiping
　　4.扫散法 33
　　4.Sweeping
　　5.拘法 33
　　5.Canceling
　　6.勒法 34
　　6.Tweezering
　　7.捋顺法 34
　　7.Stripping and Conforming
　　8.拂法、刮法 34
　　8.Skimming and Scraping

第三节　摩揉类手法 35
SECTION 3　CATEGORY OF CIRCULAR-MOVING MANIPULATIONS

一、代表手法　摩法 35
　　Principal Techniques of Circular-moving Manipulations: Circular-rubbing
　　1.指摩法 35
　　1.Circular-rubbing with the fingers
　　2.掌摩法 36
　　2.Circular-rubbing with the palm

二、摩法的衍化 37
　　Evolution of Circular-rubbing

目录

Contents

1. 揉法 37
1. Kneading
2. 运法 39
2. Transporting
3. 旋推法 40
3. Circular-pushing

三、复合手法　按揉法 40
Compound Manipulation: Pressing-Kneading

第四节　推㨰类手法 42
SECTION 4 CATEGORY OF PUSHING-ROLLING MANIPULATIONS

一、代表手法1　一指禅推法 42
Principal Techniques 1 of Pushing-Rolling Manipulations: Dhyana-Thumb-Pushing

二、一指禅推法的衍化
Evolution of Dhyana-Thumb-Pushing

1. 偏峰推 45
1. Thumb-pushing with the side tip
2. 蝴蝶双飞 46
2. Couple flying butterflies
3. 屈指推 46
3. Pushing with flexed thumb
4. 双手交叉扶持推 46
4. Dhyana-thumb-pushing supported by the crossed hands
5. 单手扶持推 47
5. Thumb-pushing supported by single hand
6. 推摩法 47
6. Dhyana-thumb-pushing and Circular-rubbing
7. 缠法 47
7. Twining

三、代表手法2　㨰法 48
Principal Techniques 2 of Pushing-Rolling Manipulation: Rolling

四、㨰法的衍化 50
Evolution of Rolling

1. 掌指关节㨰法 50
1. Rolling with the metacarpo-phalangeal joints
2. 滚法 50
2. Rolling with the proximal interphalangeal joints

第五节　捏拿类手法 53
SECTION 5 CATEGORY OF PINCHING-GRASPING MANIPULATIONS

一、代表手法　捏法 53
Principal Techniques of Pinching-Grasping Manipulations:Pinching
   1.拇示指捏 53
   1.Pinching with the thumb and index finger
   2.拇示中指捏 54
   2.Pinching with the thumb, the index and middle fingers

二、捏法的衍化 55
Evolution of Pinching
   1.拿法 55
   1.Grasping
   2.抓法 56
   2.Seizing
   3.弹筋法 56
   3.Plucking tendon
   4.挤法 57
   4.Squeezing
   5.扯法 57
   5.Tearing
   6.拧法 58
   6.Twisting
   7.挪法 58
   7.Shifting
   8.合法 58
   8.Concentrating

三、复合手法 59
Compound-manipulations
   1.捏揉法、拿揉法 59
   1.Pinching-kneading, Grasping-kneading
   2.捻法 59
   2.Holding-kneading
   3.搓法 59
   3.Rubbing with two palms

第六节　振动类手法 60
SECTION 6　CATEGORY OF VIBRATING MANIPULATIONS

一、代表手法　振法 60
Principal Techniques of Vibrating Manipulations: Vibrating
   1.指振法 61
   1.Vibrating with the fingers
   2.掌振法 61
   2.Vibrating with the palm

二、振法的衍化　摆法 62
Evolution of the Vibrating: Waving

目录 / Contents

三、复合手法 63
Compound Manipulations
    1.提颤法 63
    1.Lifting-trembling
    2.荡法 63
    2.Swinging
    3.对掌振法 64
    3.Concentrating-Vibrating

第七节 叩击类手法 64
SECTION 7 CATEGORY OF KNOCKING MANIPULATIONS

一、代表手法 击法 65
Principal Techniques of the Knocking Manipulation: Knocking
    1.拳背击 65
    1.Knocking with the fist back
    2.捶击 65
    2.Thumping
    3.掌根击 66
    3.Knocking with the palm heel
    4.掌侧击 66
    4.Knocking with the palm edge
    5.棒击 66
    5.Knocking with the stick

二、击法的衍化 67
Evolution of Knocking
    1.叩法 67
    1.Tapping
    2.拍法 68
    2.Patting
    3.啄法 69
    3.Pecking
    4.弹法 69
    4.Flicking

第八节 托插类手法 70
SECTION 8 CATEGORY OF SUPPORTING-INSERTING MANIPULATIONS

一、代表手法 托法 70
Principal Techniques of Supporting-inserting Manipulations: Supporting
二、其他手法 71
Other manipulations
    1.插法 71

  1.Inserting
 2.勾法 71
  2.Hooking

第九节 环摇类手法 72
SECTION 9 CATEGORY OF ROTATING MANIPULATIONS

一、摇颈 73
 Rotating of the Neck
 1.坐位摇颈 73
  1.Rotating of the neck in sitting position
 2.卧位摇颈 73
  2.Rotating of the neck in supine position

二、摇肩 74
 Rotating of the Shoulder
 1.托肘摇肩 74
  1.Rotating of the shoulder while supporting the elbow
 2.握手摇肩 75
  2.Rotating of the shoulder while holding the hand
 3.抡摇肩关节 75
  3.Rotating of the shoulder like windmill
 4.卧位展筋摇肩 77
  4.Rotating of the shoulder for stretching the tendon in supine position
 5.卧位点揉摇肩 77
  5.Rotating of the shoulder while kneading in supine position

三、摇肘 78
 Rotating of the Elbow

四、摇腕 78
 Rotating of the Wrist

五、摇指 79
 Rotating of the Finger

六、摇腰 79
 Rotating of the Lumbus
 1.坐位摇腰 79
  1.Rotating of the lumbus in sitting position
 2.卧位摇腰 80
  2.Rotating of the lumbus in supine position

七、摇髋 80
 Rotating of the Hip

八、摇膝 81
 Rotating of the Knee

九、摇踝 81
 Rotating of the Ankle

目录 Contents

第十节 推扳类手法 82
SECTION 10 CATEGORY OF THE THRUSTING-WRENCHING MANIPULATIONS

一、扳颈 82
Wrenching of the Neck

1. 前屈展筋扳颈 82
1. Flexion-wrenching of the neck for stretching the tendon
2. 侧屈展筋扳颈 83
2. Lateral flexion-wrenching of the neck for stretching the tendon
3. 侧屈推扳法 83
3. Lateral flexion-thrusting-wrenching of the neck
4. 卧位侧屈推扳法 84
4. Lateral flexion-thrusting-wrenching of the neck in prone position
5. 卧位侧屈牵引扳 85
5. Lateral flexion-wrenching of the neck under traction in supine position
6. 坐位斜扳法 85
6. Oblique-wrenching of the neck in sitting position
7. 卧位斜扳法 86
7. Oblique-wrenching of the neck in supine position
8. 卧位侧屈旋转扳 86
8. Lateral flexion-rotation-wrenching of the neck in supine position
9. 坐位摇扳法 87
9. Rotating-wrenching of the neck in sitting position
10. 旋转定位扳法 88
10. Rotation-wrenching of the neck on selected site
11. 俯卧位牵引旋转扳 88
11. Rotation-wrenching of the neck under traction in prone position

二、扳肩 91
Wrenching of the Shoulder

1. 前举扳肩 91
1. Flexion-wrenching of the shoulder
2. 外展扳肩 91
2. Abduction-wrenching of the shoulder
3. 内收扳肩 91
3. Adduction-wrenching of the shoulder
4. 后弯扳肩 92
4. Posterior bending-wrenching of the shoulder
5. 旋转扳肩 93
5. Rotation-wrenching of the shoulder

三、扳肘 98
Wrenching of the Elbow

1. 屈曲扳肘 98
1. Flexion-wrenching of the elbow

2.桡骨头半脱位复位法 99
2.Reduction of the radius head subluxation
3.伸肘旋前扳 99
3.Extension-pronation-wrenching of the elbow

四、扳胸
Wrenching of the Thoracic Vertebrae

1.按背扳肩法 100
1.Wrenching the shoulder while pressing on the dorsum
2.按背扳骨盆法 101
2.Wrenching the pelvis while pressing on the dorsum
3.旋转定位扳 101
3.Rotation-wrenching of the thoracic-vertebrae on selected site
4.双人旋转定位扳 102
4.Rotation-wrenching of the thoracic-lumbar vertebrae on selected site by two manipulators
5.侧屈扳法 102
5.Lateral flexion-wrenching of the thoracic vertebra
6.坐位推扳法 103
6.Thrusting-wrenching of the thoracic vertebra in sitting position

五、扳腰
Wrenching of the Lumbar Vertebrae

1.斜扳法 104
1.Oblique wrenching of the lumbar vertebrae
2.改良斜扳法 105
2.Modified oblique wrenching of lumbar vertebrae
3.旋转定位扳法 107
3.Rotation-wrenching of lumbar vertebrae on selected site
4.按腰扳腿法 108
4.Wrenching leg while pressing on lumbar
5.后伸扳腰法 109
5.Wrenching of lumbar vertebrae by extending lower extrimity

六、扳骶髂关节
Wrenching of Sacroiliac Joint

1.骶髂关节斜扳法 110
1.Oblique wrenching of sacroiliac joint
2.改良斜扳法 111
2.Modified oblique wrenching of sacroiliac joint
3.直腿抬高扳法 112
3.Wrenching of sacroiliac joint by straight lifting leg
4.拽腿扳法 113
4.Wrenching of sacroiliac joint by pulling flexed lower extremity
5.坐位屈膝屈髋扳法 113
5.Wrenching of sacroiliac joint by flexing the knee and the hip joints in sitting position
6.按骶扳腿法 114

6.Wrenching leg while pressing on sacrum

七、扳髋 114
Wrenching of the Hip
 1.小儿髋关节错缝复位手法 114
 1.Reduction of hip joint subluxation in children
 2.成人髋关节错缝复位手法 115
 2.Reduction of hip joint subluxation in adults
 3."4"字扳法 116
 3.Wrenching of hip joint as constrained Patrick's test

八、扳膝 118
Wrenching of Knee
 1.屈膝扳法 118
 1.Flexion-wrenching of knee
 2.伸膝扳法 118
 2.Extension-wrenching of knee
 3.屈膝推扳法 118
 3.Thrusting-wrenching of knee in flexion position

九、扳足踝 120
Wrenching of Ankle and Foot
 1.扳踝关节 120
 1.Wrenching of ankle
 2.距下关节错位复位法 121
 2.Reduction of the subtalar joint subluxation
 3.距舟关节错位复位法 122
 3.Reduction of the talonavicular joint subluxation

第十一节 背顶类手法 123
SECTION 11   CATEGORY OF COUNTERWORKING MANIPULATIONS

一、背法 124
Carrying on Back
 1.背法 124
 1.Carrying on back
 2.侧背法 125
 2.Lateral carrying on back

二、对抗复位法 125
Antagonistic Reduction of Thoracic Vertebrae

三、顶法 126
Counterworking
 1.仰卧位顶法 126
 1.Counterworking in supine position
 2.坐位顶法 126
 2.Counterworking in sitting position
 3.立位顶法 127
 3.Counterworking in standing position

四、踩跷法 128
Stepping

第十二节 拔伸类手法 129
SECTION 12 CATEGORY OF PULLING-STRETCHING MANIPULATIONS

一、拔颈项 129
Pulling of the Neck
1. 虎口托颌拔颈法 129
1. Pulling of the neck by supporting jaw with thumb web
2. 前臂托颌拔颈法 130
2. Pulling of the neck by supporting jaw with forearm
3. 卧位拔颈法 130
3. Pulling of the neck in supine position

二、拔伸上肢 131
Pulling of Upper Limb
1. 夹腕拔肩法 131
1. Pulling shoulder while clipping wrist
2. 膝顶拔肩法 131
2. Pulling shoulder while supporting armpit with knee
3. 肩顶拔肩法 131
3. Pulling shoulder while supporting armpit with shoulder
4. 腕关节拔伸法 132
4. Pulling of wrist
5. 指间关节拔伸法 132
5. Pulling of interphalangeal joint

三、拔伸躯干 132
Pulling of Trunk

四、拔伸下肢 133
Pulling of Lower Limb
1. 骶髂关节、髋关节拔伸法 133
1. Pulling of sacroiliac joint and hip joint
2. 踝关节拔伸法 134
2. Pulling of ankle joint

第十三节 端提类手法 134
SECTION 13 CATEGORY OF LIFTING MANIPULATIONS

一、端提头颈 135
Lifting of Neck
1. 背后操作 135
1. Lifting of neck manipulated behind patient
2. 前面操作 135
2. Lifting of neck manipulated in front of patient

二、端提胸胁 136

目录

Lifting of Thorax and Ribs

三、端提腰椎 136
Lifting of Lumbar Vertebrae

第十四节 抖动类手法 137
SECTION 14 CATEGORY OF SHAKING MANIPULATIONS

一、抖上肢 138
Shaking of Upper Limb

二、抖腕部 138
Shaking of Wrist

三、抖下肢 139
Shaking of Lower Limb

四、抖腰 139
Shaking of Waist

第三章 推拿操作常规
CHAPTER 3 THE ROUTINE TECHNIQUES OF TUINA

一、头面部操作常规 141
The Routine Techniques on Head and Facial Regions

二、颈项部操作常规 144
The Routine Techniques on Neck and Nape Regions

三、肩部操作常规 146
The Routine Techniques on the Shoulder Region

四、肘部操作常规 148
The Routine Techniques on the Elbow Region

五、腕手操作常规 150
The Routine Techniques on the Wrist and the Hand Regions

六、腰背部操作常规 152
The Routine Techniques on the Back Region

七、胸腹部操作常规 154
The Routine Techniques on the Thoracoabdominal Regions

八、髋臀部操作常规 156
The Routine Techniques on the Buttock and the Hip Regions

九、膝部操作常规 159
The Routine Techniques on the Knee Region

十、足踝部操作常规 161
The Routine Techniques on the Ankle and the Foot Regions

第一章 概 论

CHAPTER 1 INTRODUCTION

手法是推拿治病的基本手段,也是人类最早掌握的医疗方法之一。相传,我国上古神农时代(约公元前3000年)名医僦贷季就掌握了按摩技术治疗疾病。世界各国古代文明也是如此。例如,16世纪欧洲探险家在游记中提到,波利尼西亚群岛的原始土著居民虽然还不知道药物治疗方法,却利用一种独特的外治法来减轻病痛。当土人患病时,就俯卧在地上,让小孩不断地在其背上来回踩踏。通过这一方法,往往能使患者很快感到病情好转。土人以为,小孩不断地踩踏背部将驱使鬼魂逃离患者躯体。但科学的解释是,小孩身体的重力,作用于背部督脉与两侧膀胱经,能激发经络系统的调整作用,治疗疾病。

The manipulation is the main therapeutic procedure of Tuina, which is also one of the earliest therapies in human history. According to ancient works of China, as early as the Shennong era(about 3000 B.C.), the famous physician Jiu Daiji held this technique to cure diseases. So did other ancient civilizations on the world. For example, it was written in European explorers' travel notes of the 16th century that the primitive tribes lived in Polynesia archipelago used a unique external therapy to relieve sufferers though they didn't know other treatments. If a native was ill, the patient lies prostrately on the ground and a child stepped on his back to and fro. In this way, the illness was often relieved or removed. They believed that the child could drive the evil out of the body. But the science explanation is that the force of the child's step acted on the Du and the Bladder Channels on the back. The latter then adjust all the life functions to remove pathological changes, or recovered from diseases.

所谓手法，是指为了医疗和保健目的，操作者用手或身体其他部位刺激人体体表或活动肢体的规范化技巧动作。由于刺激方式、强度、时间的不同，形成了许多动作不同的基本手法，如按法、拿法、推法；把两个以上的基本手法结合起来操作，就成为复合手法，如按揉法、推摩法、捏揉法；把一连串动作组合起来操作，并冠以特定的名称，就称为复式操作法，如打马过天河、黄蜂入洞、赤凤摇头。

Manipulations are defined those standardized skillful actions in which the manipulator stimulate body surface or move the limbs or trunks of the patient with their hands or other body parts for medical and healthy goal. Owing to the differences in stimulation patterns, intensities and times, there are a lot of different elementary manipulations such as pressing, grasping and pushing etc. Combined with two or more elementary manipulations, they become compound manipulations such as pressing kneading. Composed a serial actions in turn and given specific terms, they are called as complex manipulative programs, as "riding horse across heaven river", "Wasp entering cavity" and "Red phoenix rotating head" etc.

推拿手法是一种技能，是一种高级的肢体运动形式，不能与日常生活中的肢体随意动作相提并论。推拿手法虽然来源于人类的日常生活动作，如推、拿、按、压、揉、捏等，但手法的直接作用对象是人体活组织，手法治疗的中介是经络系统，手法作用部位又常存在各种病理改变，故手法必须符合特定的技术要求，遵循严格的操作规范，掌握操作技能，使手法既能对经络系统发挥最大的激发作用，又不致对人体局部组织造成伤害，取得最佳的治疗效果。中医推拿历来重视手法技能在治疗中的作用，《医宗金鉴·正骨心法要旨》云："伤有轻重，而手法各有所异，其痊可之迟速及遗留残疾与否，皆关乎手法之所施得宜。"推拿治病主要靠手法技能的运用，而不是靠力气，更不是靠粗暴蛮力。临床常见到有些患者经非专业医师"推拿治疗"后，不仅原有的病痛没有消除，反而造成皮肤破损、皮下瘀斑，甚至引起严重医疗事故的发生。不讲究操作技能的动作决不是手法。

Tuina manipulation is high-skilled techniques or expertly movement of the body. They should not be regarded as the casual action of everyday life, though they originated from those actions such as push, grasp, press and knead etc. Their direct impact object is the living tissue of the body, where is usually pathologically changed. And their intermediary is the channel system. Therefore, the manipulation must be specially required in technique and in clinic application. Only the high-skill manipulation and the properly selected indication, will Tuina promote the self-adjusting function of the channel system and attain good curative effect, without harming the local tissues of the body. Tuina of Traditional Chinese Medicine has been putting special emphasis on the role of manipulation in clinic practice. It was pointed out that, in the ancient classic book *Yi Zong Jin Jian*, the chapter "Zheng Gu Xin Fa Yao Zhi," "There are different manipulations and traumas serious or not. Therefore that the trauma recovered quick or slow, complete or not, all depends on if the manipulations are suitable or not." The curative effect of Tuina is relied on the manipulative skill instead of the force and says nothing of violence. It is often seen in clinical experiences that some patient's sufferings are not relieved after "Tuina therapy" offered by nonprofessional persons. Instead, their skins were abrades, their subcutaneous tissues injured. Even more, seriously medical accidents were happened. The action without special techniques is definitely not Tuina manipulations.

第一节 手法的分类
SECTION 1 CLASSIFICATION OF THE MANIPULATIONS

中医推拿素以历史悠久,流派众多,手法丰富,技巧性强,适应证广,疗效显著而著称于世。根据目前统计,我国有文字记载的推拿手法已有200余种,而流传于民间尚未定型的手法可能更多。手法虽然繁多,但可以根据其外力作用方式而划分为两门,即《内经》所言的"按"和"蹻"。根据唐代医家王冰的注释,"按"为"抑按皮肉","蹻"为"捷举手足"。前者的手法力直接作用于接触部位,而后者的外力间接作用于远离接触部位的关节、肌肉、筋膜。每一门手法又可根据动作特点而分为若干类,每一类手法又包括若干种基本手法,每一基本手法还可根据其接触部位、动作变化而分为若干种变法。若从手法的主要作用途径分类,则可以分为刺激性手法、矫正性手法和松动性手法。各类手法间的相互关系如图1。

Tuina of traditional Chinese Medicine is famous for its long history, numerous schools, plentiful manipulations, high skills, broad indication range and outstanding curative effects. According to present statistics, there are more than 200 Tuina manipulations described in books in China. And there are still more manipulations prevailed in folk. Although the manipulations are numerous, they can be classed into 2 phylum on the basis of the action of external force. They are the "pressing" and the "rectifying" written in the ancient classic book *Nei Jing*. The "pressing" means to restrain, to press skin and muscle while the "Rectifying" means to move limb quickly, in the light of the famous scholar Wang Bing who lived in the Tang Dynasty. The force of the former impacts directly on the local tissues where are contacted by the manipulator's hand, but the force of the latter transmitted to the distant joint, muscles, tendons and so on. Each phylum can be divided into some categories too, according to their motion features. And each category contains several elementary manipulations. Even more, on the basis of their touch parts and motion changes, each elementary manipulation is constituted by some varieties. If the manipulations are classified according to their main effect processes, they can be divided into stimulating manipulations(or so called reflection manipulations abroad), rectifying manipulations and mobilizing manipulations. The relation among the various manipulations is showed below.

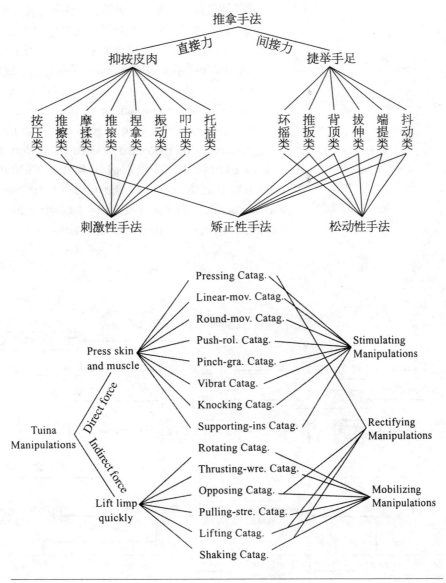

图1 推拿手法谱系
Fig. 1 The Pedigree of Tuina Manipulations

第二节 推拿手法的作用途径
SECTION 2 EFFECTING PROCESSES OF THE MANIPULATIONS

推拿手法的本质是一种外力,手法外力既可直接引起关节位置的改变,肌肉、筋膜等软组织的形变、撕裂而纠正人体病理状态,治愈疾病。但更重要的是,手法外力作为一种刺激因素,激活了经络系统的调整功能,使机体趋于康复。

The essence of Tuina manipulations is external force. The force of the manipulations can either directly correct the subluxation or disalignments of the joints, cause the soft tissues to be deformed and the adhesion separated so as to redress the pathological status and cure disease. More important is that, the force of the manipulations, as a stimulate factor, activates adjusting function of the channel system to make rehabilitation.

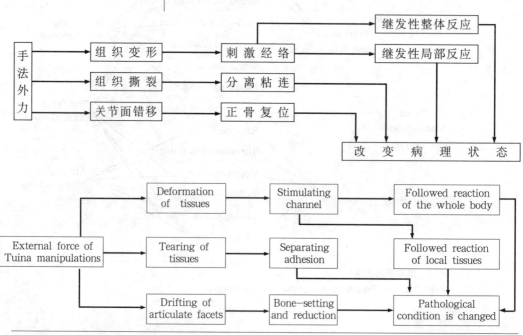

图2 推拿手法主要作用途径
Fig. 2 Main effecting processes of manipulation

第三节　推拿手法的技术要求
SECTION 3 TECHNICAL REQUIREMENTS OF TUINA MANIPULATIONS

1. 刺激性手法的技术要求

抑按皮肉门手法中，大多数为刺激性手法，刺激性手法并不是以本身直接的力改变人体的病理状态而发挥治疗效应，而是手法作用于经络系统，再通过经络系统的中介，激发人体固有的调整与自愈功能，才能防病治病。故刺激性手法必须符合持久、有力、均匀、柔和、深透等技术要求。

1. Technical requirement of stimulating manipulations

Most manipulation of the "Pressing skin and muscle" belongs to the stimulating manipulation. The stimulating manipulations don't directly relay on their force to remove illness and make recovery. But they act on the channel system and then through its medium to promote the intrinsic adjusting and self-curing functions of the life to prevent or to heal disease. So the stimulating manipulations must tally with endurable, forceful, regular, gentle and penetrable requirements.

所谓持久，是指手法能严格按照特定操作规范持续运用一段时间而不走样，使手法的刺激量积累到临界点，足以推动经络系统的调整作用，改变病理状态。例如，小儿推拿的"推三关"和"退六腑"手法对某些病情严重的患儿必须连续操作半小时以上才能发挥显著的解表发汗或退热作用。所谓有力，就是指手法应具有恰当的力量。在一定的范围内，手法力的大小与对经络系统的刺激强度成正比，但超过这个限度，反而造成组织损伤，或成为一种超限抑制信号。手法力的大小也并不是固定不变的，必须根据施术部位、病理特点、患者体质等具体情况而调整力的大小。根据临床具体情况而施加恰当的手法力，需经过长期的实践才能掌握。所谓"均匀"，是指手法动作要有节奏性，速度不可时快时慢，压力不可时轻时重。图3为一指禅推法动力测试曲线记录，图表中曲线波形高度、宽度及形态显示非常一致。所谓"柔和"，是指手法的用力方式，平稳而缓慢变化的力要比急剧变化的暴发力柔和，以柔软易变形的掌面着力要比以坚硬而不易变形的骨突着力柔和。所谓"深透"，是指通过运用各种富于技巧性的手法，降低人体活组织的张力，减少对外力传递的阻抗而使手法作用达到组织深层。

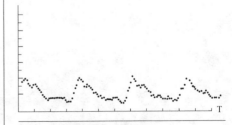

图3　一指禅推法动力测试曲线
Fig. 3　Dynamic measuring curve of Dhyana thumb pushing

The so-called "endurable" means that the manipulations must be correctly handled for a long time according to specific rules. Thus the quantity of stimulation of the manipulation will accumulate to a critical point, which is big enough to push forward the adjusting function of the channel system, so as to improve pathological status. For example, "Pushing Sanguan" and " Retreating Liufu" in the Pediatric Tuina clinic must be manipulated for more than half an hour, only then can it exert a remarkable effect of diaphoresis or antifebrile on some serious infant patients. The so-called " forceful" means that the manipulations must keep in suitable force. In a given range, the quantity of manipulation force is direct proportion with the stimulating intensity to the channel system. But if it is over the limit, the force can injure the tissues or become a over-limitation suppressive message to weaken the function of channel. The quantity of manipulation force is also not fixed. It must be adjusted according to the acting parts, the pathological features, the patient's constitutions and so on. To apply a suitable force on the basis of clinical conditions can be held only through a long time practice. The so-called "regular" means that the motion of manipulations must have rhythm. The velocity can't be sometimes fast, sometimes slow. The force can't be sometimes heavy, sometimes light. The Fig.3 is a measure curve of "Dhyana-pushing" with thumb. The height, the width and the pattern of the curve show identical. The so-called "gentle" refers to the patterns of delivering force. The force, which is varied smoothly and slowly, is gentler than those varied violently and quickly. The touch styles with a soft flexible tissue such as palm are gentler than those with a hard, inflexible tissue such as bone. The so-called "penetrable" refers to apply all skillful manipulation to reduce the tension of human living tissues so that the resistance of the tissues would be cut down and the manipulation force could act into deep tissue.

2. 矫正性、松动性手法的技术要求

矫正性手法和松动性手法统称"关节运动性手法"。典型的

关节运动的各种范围如图4。

2. Technical requirements of rectifying and mobilizing manipulations

　　Rectifying and mobilizing manipulations are also called as "manipulations of joint motion". All ranges of typical joint motion are as Fig. 4.

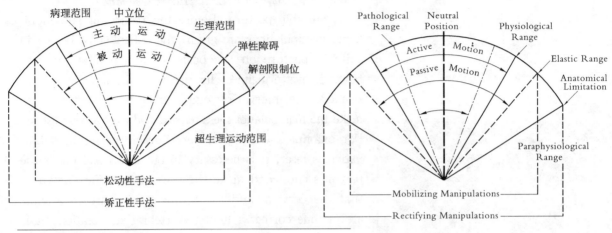

图4　关节运动范围与手法关系
Fig. 4　The Relation of joint motion range and manipulations

　　矫正性手法和松动性手法通常作用于已存在运动障碍的关节，而手法的完成又必须突破关节的病理运动限制范围或生理运动限制范围，必然刺激病变组织，引起疼痛及保护性反应。此外，由于病理产物的刺激，关节运动肌群处于痉挛状态，使手法完成所需要的被动运动幅度或关节面分离运动难以实现。故矫正性、松动性手法必须遵循以下要求。

　　In general, the rectifying and mobilizing manipulations act on those joints that have been suffered from motion limitation. And the accomplishments of manipulation have to break the pathological limit position or physiological limit position. So they certainly excite the pathologically changed tissues and give rise to pain and protective reaction. Beside, due to the stimulation of pathological products, the motion muscles of the joint are in spasm situation. It is difficult for the physician to fulfill the necessary range of passive movement and facet shift of the joint. So the rectifying and mobilizing manipulations must abide by the following requirements.

(1)体位适当：在运用矫正性手法和松动性手法前，必须按照人体生物力学原理，给被施术者摆好合适的体位，使病变关节肌肉松弛，关节间隙增大，减少手法操作中的阻力，易于手法完成。如矫正上胸段椎骨错缝时，胸前垫一软枕，头颈略下垂，使颈椎和胸椎处于同一弧线上。又如矫正腰椎椎骨错缝时，调整上身扭转的幅度和下肢屈髋的角度，使脊柱扭转中心正好落在错位的运动单元上，手法就容易完成。

(1)Suitable posture：Before the rectifying and mobilizing manipulations are given, the patient must be put in suitable posture on the basis of human anatomy and biomechanics principles. In this way, the muscles will be relaxed, the interval of joint will be broadened so as to make the manipulations less resisted and easy accomplished. For example, when a upper thoracic vertebral subluxation is reset, it is necessary to put a soft pad under the patient's chest and make the neck slightly flex down so that the cervical and the thoracic spine are in a same arc. If one correct a lumbar vertebral subluxation, it is better to adjust the right rotation range of the spine and suitable flexion degree of hip. Thus the twisting center of the spine is just located at subluxation segment and the manipulation is controlled easy.

(2)用力平稳、轻巧、短促、随发随收：矫正性手法和松动性手法的操作过程一般分为两个阶段，先平稳地将关节运动到某一限制位，然后作一轻巧、短促的突发动作，扩大关节运动幅度，随即停止用力，使关节恢复中立位。

(2)Smoothly, lightly, sleight briefly controlled：The manipulative course is usually divided into 2 phases. First, the joint is moved to a limited situation smoothly and slowly. Second, a light, ingenious, controlled and sudden thrusting is done to expand the range of joint motion. As soon as the thrusting is done, one must stop it and regain the joint in neutral status.

(3)把握正确的用力方向：手法操作时，必须考虑到关节面的形态，关节瞬时运动中心的位置，关节面互相错移的方向而把握正确的用力方向。否则，难以完成手法目标。例如，骶髂关节错位有后错(髂后上棘隆凸)和前错(髂后上棘低陷)两型，前者应按髂后上棘向前外下用力，按骶骨下端向上方用力；而后者应按坐骨结节向前外上用力，按骶骨上端向前下方用力。若用力方向不对，就不可能达到复位的目的。

(3)Correct direction of exerting force: During the manipulative process, one must consider about those things such as the shape of joint facet, the instantaneous center of joint motion and the direction at which the two joint surfaces will move along, in order to hold the correct force direction of manipulation. Otherwise, it is impossible to achieve the goal of the manipulation. For instance, there are posterior subluxation and anterior subluxation at sacroiliac joint. For the former, one should thrust the posterior superior iliac spine directed anterior laterior and inferior, and the lower end of sacrum directed anterior superior in the same time. But for the latter, it is suitable to thrust the ischium directed anterior laterior and superior, and the upper end of sacrum directed anterior inferior in the same time. If the direction controlled wrong, it is very difficult to restore the subluxation.

第二章 推拿手法

CHAPTER 2 TUINA MANIPULATIONS

第一节 按压类手法

SECTION 1 CATEGORY OF PRESSING MANIPULATIONS

所谓按压类手法是指把操作者的掌、指或身体其他部位置于患者体表后,沿体表垂直方向向深部用力的一类手法(图5)。

The category of pressing manipulations is referred to those actions in which the manipulator puts his palm, finger or other parts of the body on the patient's body surface and delivers force at the vertical direction to the body surface(Fig.5).

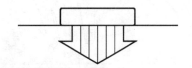

图5 按压类手法模式图
Fig. 5 Model of Category of Pressing Manipulations

一、代表手法 按法
Principal Techniques of Pressing Manipulations: Pressing

按法以拇指指端或指腹接触,为指按法;用掌根部接触,称掌按法。既可单手操作,又可两手相叠,增加按压力量,协同操作。

Those pressings in which the manipulator presses on the patient's bodies with thumb tip or thumbprint called as pressing with the thumb, while those with palm heel is called as pressing with the palm. They may be done with single hand, or with two lapped hands in coordination to strengthen the pressing force.

推 拿 手 法

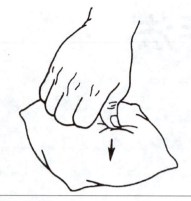

图6 指按法
Fig. 6 Pressing with thumb

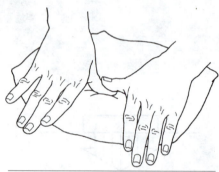

图7 叠指按
Fig. 7 Pressing with lapped thumbs

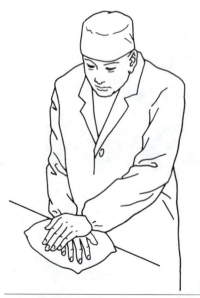

图8 掌按法
Fig. 8 Pressing with Palm

1. 指按法

拇指伸直，其余四指自然弯曲，示指与拇指相靠，助拇指指力；用前臂的力量，逐渐向下按压，用力由轻而重，使刺激充分深透到机体组织深部后，逐渐减轻压力，再重复以上的按压过程(图6)。欲增加按压力量，可将另一手拇指重叠于指骨间关节上，两指协同向下按压(图7)。

1. Pressing with thumb

The operator extends the thumb with his four fingers flexed naturally and the index finger leaned against the thumb to enhance its strength, the manipulator extends the thumb and puts it at a point. Then applies forearms power to press downward gradually. The force is varied from slight to heavy until the stimulation fully penetrated into the deep tissues, then it is reduced. This process is repeated for several times (Fig.6). If you want to strengthen pressing force, one can overlap other thumb on the interphalangeal joint of the thumb to press down coordinately (Fig.7).

指按法接触面积小而集中，刺激强弱容易控制，适合于全身各部的穴位与反应点、压痛点操作，具有较好的止痛作用，常用于各种痛证的治疗。

The contact area of pressing with the thumb is small and concentrated. Its stimulating intensity can be controlled easily. So it is adapted for acting on all the acupoints, reflecting points and trigger points. It has strong analgesic effect and is often used to treat pain syndromes.

2. 掌按法

掌按法以两手操作居多。操作时，手指自然伸直，腕关节背伸，一手掌根部接触体表，另一手掌重叠其上，上肢伸直；然后以肩部或躯干发力，逐渐增加按压力量，使力沿伸直的上肢纵轴传达到按压部位，待刺激充分深透后再逐渐减小按压力量。重复以上操作(图8)。

2. Pressing with palm

Two hands partner is more often seen than single-hand manner. During the manipulation, the manipulator extends the fingers naturally and the wrist slightly, and puts the hand heel on patient's body and overlaps the other hand on it. The force generated by the shoulder or the trunk is transmitted to the pressing areas along the straightening upper limbs. The pressing force is increased until the stimulation is fully and deeply penetrated, then it is reduced gradually. The above action is repeated for several times(Fig.8).

掌按法按压力量大，接触面积也大，适用于腰背部、臀部、大腿、小腿和肩部操作，具有较好的放松痉挛肌组织的作用，常用于治疗急慢性腰腿痛、肩关节周围炎等病证。

The force of pressing with palm is strong, its contact area is also big. It is suitable for acting on the back, the buttocks, the thigh, the shank and the shoulder. It has a good effect to relax convulsive muscles and is usually applied to cure acute and chronic lumbar-leg pains and scapulohumeral periarthritis.

二、按法的衍化
Evolution of Pressings

1. 肘压法

按是指手法的动作形态，压是指手法所引起的压缩效应，故通常按压混称。若严格区分两者，则"按"偏于动，"压"偏于静；按的压力持续时间短，压的刺激持续时间长；按的压力小，刺激轻；压的力量大，刺激强。用肘部按压习惯称为"肘压法"，肘压操作时，肘关节屈曲，以肘尖置体表某部，用上肢与躯干发力，垂直向下按压。肘压法刺激强烈，一般仅用于肌肉发达厚实的下腰部、臀部操作，治疗顽固性腰腿痛、腰肌僵硬等病证。

1. Compressing with the elbow

In Chinese, pressing refers to the motive pattern of manipulation while compressing refers to the effect caused by the manipulation. So the pressing and the compressing are often lumped together in Tuina books. If you want to strictly distinguish them, the "pressing" is inclined to motion, while the "compressing" is inclined to static. The duration time of the pressing is shorter than that of the compressing. The force and the stimulation intensity of the former are also slighter than those of the compressing. The manipulation in which the elbow is

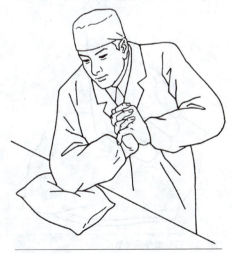

图9 肘压法
Fig. 9 Compressing with the elbow

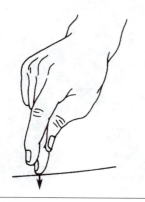

图10 中指点法

Fig. 10 Pointing with the middle finger

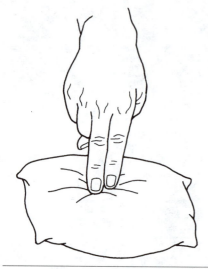

图11 剑指点法

Fig. 11 Pointing with the "sword fingers"

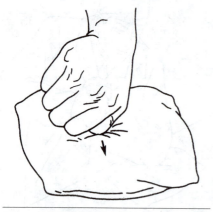

图12 拇指指骨间关节点

Fig. 12 Pointing with interphalangeal joint of the thumb

used to press is used to being named for compressing with elbow. When you exercise compressing with elbow, you should flex the elbow joint, put the elbow tip on patient's body, and then deliver force from shoulder and trunk muscles to compress downward. Because its stimulation is fairly intense, it is only used on the low back and buttocks on which the muscles are well developed to cure persistent lumbar-leg pains and lumbar stiff.

2. 点法

如欲得到比指按法刺激更强的穴位刺激，则可减小按压时的接触面积，称为点法。点法有4种操作方式：①中指点：拇、示、中三指自然伸直，拇指置中指掌侧，示指置中指背侧，挟持中指助力，然后利用腕、肘、肩关节力量，以中指端点按穴位，使刺激深入组织深部，然后将手指抬起(图10)。②剑指点：示、中二指伸直成剑指，然后仿中指点操作方式，利用腕、肘、肩关节的力量，以示、中二指指端点按穴位(图11)。③拇指指骨间关节点：手握空拳，以屈曲的拇指指骨间关节骨突点按穴位(图12)。④示指指骨间关节点：手握空拳，用拇指尺侧缘抵住示指指甲，然后以屈曲的示指近侧指骨间关节骨突点按穴位(图13)。

2. Pointing

If you want to get a stronger stimulation than pressing with the thumb, you may reduce the touch area and the manipulation becomes pointing. There are four manipulative manners. The first, pointing with middle finger is manipulated as that: Extending thumb, index finger and middle finger naturally, putting the thumb against the palm side of the middle finger and the index finger against the back side to strengthen the middle finger, then the manipulator delivers power from the wrist, elbow, or shoulder joint to point and press acupoints with the tip of the middle finger. Until the stimulation penetrates into the deep tissue, then lifts the middle finger (Fig.10). The second, pointing with the "sword fingers" can be done as follows: Stretching the index and the middle fingers to form so-called "sword fingers", then the manipulator imitates the pattern of the pointing with the middle finger to deliver the power from the wrist, the elbow, or the shoulder to point and press acupoints with the tip of the fingers (Fig.11). The third, pointing with the interphalangeal joint of the thumb, is manipulated as that: making a hollow fist, then the manipulator points and presses acupoints with the bone bulge on back side of the interphalangeal joint of a flexed thumb (Fig. 12). The fourth, pointing with the interphalangeal joint of the index finger, may be done in this way: Making a hollow fist, supporting the index finger nail with the palm side of the thumb, then the manipulator points and presses acupoints with the bone bulge on the back side of the proximal interphalangeal joint of the flexed index finger (Fig.13).

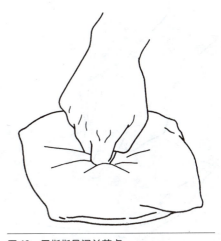

图 13 示指指骨间关节点
Fig. 13 Pointing with interphalangeal joint of the index finger

点法较按法刺激强而持续时间短，适用于骨缝关节处穴位操作及各种剧烈疼痛、瘫痪等病证的治疗，但对于一般患者，多以按法施之。

The stimulation force of pointing is stronger than that of pressing, but its duration is shorter than that of the latter. Pointing is adapted for acting on the points which situate in bone cracks and joint interval or causing severe pain and paralysis. But for common patients, pressing is more frequently used.

3. 掐法

如再缩小点按接触的面积，使刺激更为强烈尖锐，则可用指甲来按压穴位，就成为掐法(图14)。又称爪法或切法。掐法刺激强烈，常用于水沟、素髎、内关、中冲、老龙等急救穴位的操作，有开窍解痉的作用，以治疗昏迷、惊风、休克等危急症。有时为了缓解掐法所形成的锐痛，在应用掐法之后，再用揉法和之。

3. Nipping with the thumbnail

If you want even to reduce the touch area of pressing and make the stimulation stronger and sharper, you may employ the thumbnail to press acupoints and the manipulation is called as nipping with the thumbnail, or scratching or cutting. The nipping with the thumbnail has a strong stimulus, and it is often manipulated on the first-aid acupoints such as Shuigou, Suliao, Neiguan, Zhongchong and Laolong etc. Since it may resuscitate one's life and dispel epileptic attack, it is used for curing

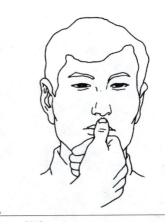

图 14 掐法
Fig. 14 Nipping with the thumbnail

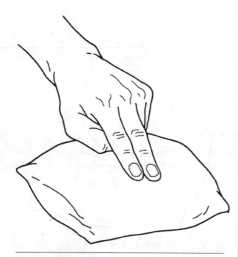

图 15 押法
Fig. 15 Touching

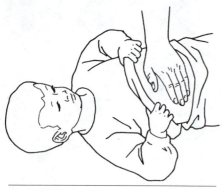

图 16 掩法、扣法
Fig. 16 Cupping, Warm covering

coma, convulsion and shock. In order to relieve acute pain caused by the nipping with the thumbnail, you may use the kneading manipulation at the nipping area after it.

4. 押法

在指按法的基础上，减轻向下按压的力量，以手指罗纹面按于穴位而不动，称押法(图15)。押法常用于探求穴位得气。

4. Touching

Based on the manipulative manner of pressing with the thumb, one reduces pressing force and keeps the fingerprint in still on acupoints. The manipulation is called as touching(Fig. 15). The touching is usually used to seek the accurate location of the acupoints and for convenience of "getting Qi".

5. 掩法、扣法

在掌按法的基础上，减轻向下按压的力量，以手掌轻按于胸腹部不动，称掩法。若按于胸腹前，先将手掌擦热，则称扣法（图16）。但在目前临床中，已不再细分，统称为掌按法。

5. Cupping, Warm covering

Based on the manipulative manner of the pressing with the palm, the pressing force being reduced and the palm being kept still on the chest or the abdomen, the manipulation becomes cupping. With two palms rubbing mutually to make the palm warm, and then the warm palm being gentle pressed on the body and keeping in still, it is named as warm covering(Fig. 16). But in present clinic application of Tuina, they have not been distinguished strictly and both called as the same name as pressing with the palm.

三、按压复位法
Pressing-Reductions

按压法是刺激性手法，按压持续时间较长而平稳。按压复位法是矫正性手法，按压突发而持续时间短暂，形成一种冲击，使骨关节面受到震动而在韧带、肌肉张力的作用下自行复位，适用于关节半脱位。

Since the pressings belong to the stimulating manipulations, the process of action is longer and smoother. While the pressing-reductions belong to the rectifying manipulations, their pressing actions last a very short time as dash. In this way, the bone and the articulate facets are shacked so that they would be restored by the tension of the ligaments and the muscles in cases of joint subluxation.

按压复位的用力方式可分为以下3种：
There are three thrust patterns in pressing-reduction manipulations.

肘关节发力：操作者以一手掌根部或尺侧缘抵住患椎棘突或横突，另一手掌根重叠按压于腕背部，肘关节微屈，身体保持不动；然后两臂作一突发有控制的动作，使肘关节伸直，在掌根部产生一幅度有限的回弹冲击力，令脊柱运动单元产生错移震动而复位（图17）。颈、胸椎复位均可使用肘关节发力方式。

The first, delivering force from the elbows. The manipulator puts one of his palm heel or ulnar side of hand on the spinous process or the transverse process of the suffered vertebra and overlaps the other palm on the wrist back, flexes the elbows slightly, and keeps the body in still. Then makes the two arms do a sudden, controlled action to stretch the elbow joints. Thus a controlled spring force is produced on the hand heel. The motion segment will produce a grinding vibration to revert its normal location (Fig.17). The reductions of cervical, thoracic vertebral subluxation may be applied with this pattern.

肩臂发力：操作者身体略侧前倾，以一手掌根按压于患椎棘突，上肢伸直；然后肩臂作一突发有控制的动作，向前下方按压（图18）。胸椎复位可采用肩臂发力方式。

The second, delivering force from the arms and the shoulders. The manipulator leans his body forward, puts a palm heel on the spinous process of the suffered vertebra and stretches the arm. Then makes the arm and the shoulder do a sudden and controlled motion to thrust at the anterior-inferior direction (Fig. 18). Reduction of

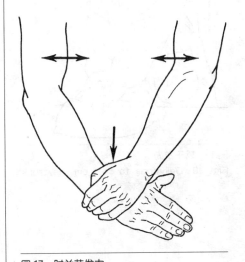

图17 肘关节发力
Fig. 17 Delivering force from the elbows

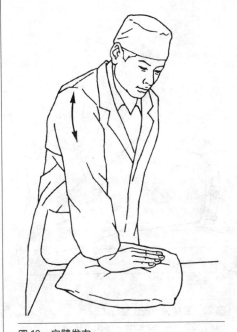

图18 肩臂发力
Fig. 18 Delivering force from the arms and the shoulders

the thoracic vertebra may be applied with this pattern.

躯干发力：操作者以一手掌根按压于一定部位上，另一手掌根重叠其上，身体略向前倾，上肢保持伸展状态，然后腰胯部作一突发有控制动作，身体下坠，利用躯干的重力和肌力，按压患者脊柱复位(图19)。本法仅应用于身体壮实者的腰椎或骶髂关节复位。

The third, delivering force from the trunk. With his trunk leaned forward, the manipulator puts one hand heel on the spinous processes, overlaps the other hand on it, and keeps his arms in stretch condition. Then makes lumbar-buttock do a sudden and controlled motion to drop down. Thus the palms thrust the spine and cause restoration with the gravitate force of the trunk and the muscular power (Fig. 19). This pattern is only used to treat those patients who suffer from the sacroiliac joint subluxation or lumbar vertebral subluxation and have strong physiques.

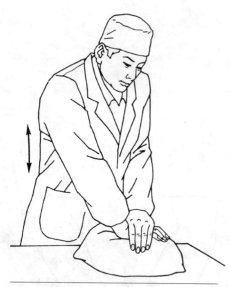

图19 躯干发力
Fig. 19 Delivering force from the trunk

具体操作如下。
Concrete Procedure as follows.

1. 寰枕关节按压复位法

患者俯卧，胸前垫枕，额部枕于相叠之两前臂上，注意保持颈椎处于前屈中立位。医生以掌根豌豆骨抵住枕外隆凸下缘向患者前上方推压，以拉开寰枕间隙，缓解枕下肌群痉挛。然后适时以肘关节发力方式，按压枕部，即可复位(图20)。本法适用于寰枕关节错位的整复。

1. Pressing-Reduction of the atlantooccipital joint

With a pad under his chest and his crossed forearms under his forehead, the patient is in prone position and keeps his cervical spine in neutrally flexed condition. The physician pushes the patient's inferior rim of the occiput directed to the patient's forehead with his pisiform of the wrist so as to broaden the atlantooccipital interval and to relax the suboccipital muscles. Then thrusts the occiput to restore the joint with the first pattern of delivering force at the suitable moment(Fig. 20). The manipulation is adapted to the subluxation of the atlantooccipital joint.

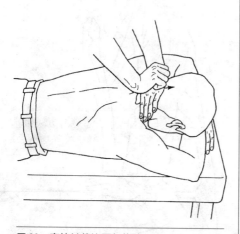

图20 寰枕关节按压复位法
Fig. 20 Pressing-reduction of the atlantooccipital joint

2. 上颈椎侧卧位按压复位法

患者侧卧，颈椎棘突偏凸侧向上，枕头厚度应适宜，以保持颈椎处于中立位。操作者以一手掌根豌豆骨抵住偏凸之颈椎棘突向脊柱中线按压，另一手虎口叉住其腕背，以拇指顶住下一颈椎骨横突向患者外前方按压；然后稍用力向下按压，使颈椎侧屈至限制位，适时用肘关节发力方式，突然加大按压力量，使颈椎运动单元两椎骨互相错移而复位(图21)。本法适用于颈4以上节段椎骨错位。

2. Pressing-reduction of the upper cervical vertebrae in laterallying position

The patient is in the lateral lying position in which the projected spinous process of the suffered cervical vertebra is upward. A suitable pillow is put under the patient's head to keep his cervical spine in neutral position. The manipulator contacts the projected spinous process with the pisiform of wrist that overlapped by the other hand and sticks against the transverse process of the lower vertebra directed at the lateroanteriorly with the thumb. Then presses the cervical spine down to make the neck be laterally bent gently until the barrier positions, and then suddenly and forcibly thrusts the spinous process and transverse process to drive the two vertebrae to be shifted oppositely and regain their normal relation (Fig.21). This manipulation is adapted to the vertebral subluxation, which are above the C4.

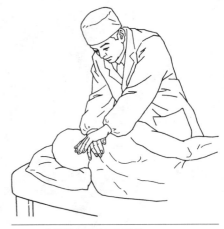

图 21　上颈椎侧卧按压复位法
Fig. 21 Pressing-reduction of the upper cervical vertebrae in lateral lying position

3. 下颈椎俯卧位按压复位法

患者俯卧，胸前垫枕，脸转向棘突偏凸侧，使颈椎保持前屈和向患侧旋转的姿势。操作者以一手掌根抵住患者枕外隆凸下缘向其前上方按压，以拉开颈椎关节间隙，缓解颈肌痉挛；另一手拇指端抵住对侧后凸之颈椎横突，向其外前上方按压，即可复位(图22)。本法适用于颈5以下节段的椎骨错缝。

3. Pressing-reduction of the lower cervical vertebrae in prone position

With a pad under his chest, the patient is in prone position and his cervical spine is kept in flexion-rotational position, in which his face is turned to the suffered side. The physician contacts the lower rim of the occiput to push it anterosuperiorly with his palm heel so as to broaden the interval of the facet joints and relax the neck

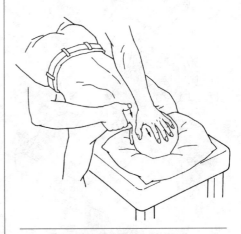

图22　下颈椎俯卧位按压复位法
Fig. 22 Pressing-reduction of the lower cervical vertebrae in prone position

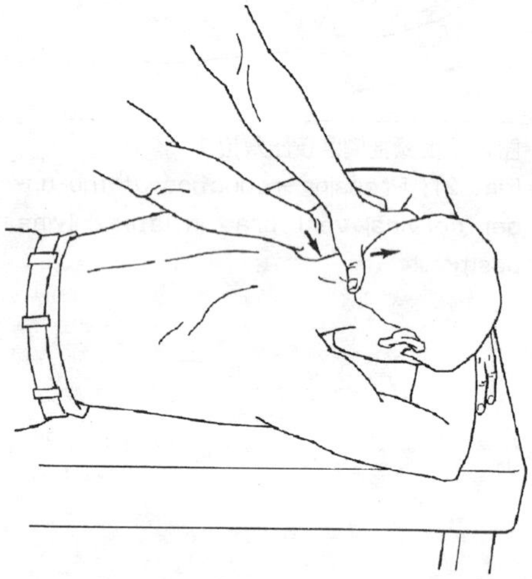

muscles and the posterior projected transverse process of the contraside with the thumb of the other hand. Then suddnly and controlly thrust the transverse process directed anterio-superiorly. Thus the vertebra is restored (Fig. 22). The manipulation is adapted to the cervical vertebral subluxation which is at the C5 or below the C5.

4. 上胸椎按压复位法

患者体位同上，保持颈椎前屈中立位，脸朝下，额部枕于相抱的两臂上，使颈椎与胸椎后凸弧度处于同一条弧线上。医生操作如上法，一手掌跟前推枕部，以牵拉颈胸肌群，另一手掌根按压后凸之胸椎横突，使之复位。本法适用于伴有斜方肌、肩胛提肌、半棘肌、颈夹肌痉挛的胸4以上节段胸椎错位，亦可用于肋椎关节复位(图23)。

4. Pressing-reduction of the upper thoracic vertebrae in prone position

The patient's position is the same as the above but the cervical spine is kept in neutral flexion position. With his forehead resting on his crossed arms, his cervical curvature and the thoracic curvature of the vertebrae is kept in a same arc. The physician's action is also like the above. With one palm heel pushing the occiput to haul the muscles that span over the cervices, thoracic vertebrae, the manipulator presses on the posterior protruded transverse process of the thoracic vertebra with the other palm and then thrusts it to make restoration. The manipulation is adapted to the vertebral subluxation of the thoracic spine which are accompanied by the trapezius, levator scapulae, splenius cervicis and semispinalis spasm and are above the T4, it can also be used to correct the subluxation of costovertebral joint (Fig. 23).

5. 上胸椎指拨复位法

患者体位与操作者操作方法同上，但医生按压胸椎横突之手改为用拇指顶住偏凸棘突向其内前方按压，使其复位(图24)。本法适用于胸4以上节段椎骨错位整复。

5. Bending-reduction of the upper thoracic vertebrae with the thumb

The patient's position and the physician's action are

图23 上胸椎按压复位法
Fig. 23 Pressing-reduction of the upper thoracic vertebrae in prone position

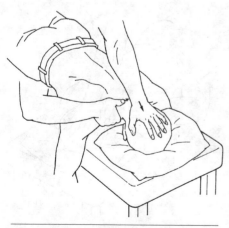

图24 上胸椎指拨复位法
Fig. 24 Bending-reduction of the upper thoracic vertebrae with the thumb

much similar to the above manipulations. But, the pressing-reduction pattern in which the physician thrusts transverse process is changed into thrusting the spinous process toward the medial anterior side of the patient with the thumb so as to cause restoration (Fig. 24). The manipulation is adapted to the subluxation of upper thoracic vertebrae above the T4.

6. 胸椎交叉按压复位法

患者俯卧。操作者将双臂交叉，以掌根豌豆骨抵住对侧同一运动单元之上下胸椎横突，嘱患者作深呼吸，待呼吸协调后，乘其吸气末期胸壁鼓起时，适时用肘关节发力，将胸椎横突向其外前方按压，使其复位（图25）。本法适用于胸4以下节段椎骨错缝。

6. Cross pressing-reduction of the thoracic vertebrae

The patient is in the prone position. The physician crosses his arms to press the two contralateral transverse processes that belong to the same motion segment but not the same vertebra with his pisiforms. Then asks the patient to take deep breath. As the patient breathes regularly and his chest wall is expanded at the end of the inhalation period, the physician thrusts the transverse process directed lateroanteriorly with the pattern of delivering force from the elbow to cause restoration (Fig. 25). The manipulation is adapted to the reduction of thoracic vertebrae subluxation below the T4.

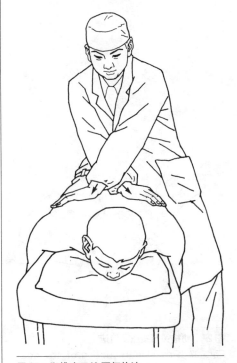

图25 胸椎交叉按压复位法
Fig. 25 Cross pressing-reduction of the thoracic vertebrae

7. 胸椎棘突下掌缘按压复位法

患者俯卧。操作者以一手掌侧缘抵住错位棘突下缘，另一手掌重叠于腕背之上；然后嘱患者深呼吸，待呼吸协调后，乘其吸气末期胸壁鼓起时，适时用肘关节发力，将棘突向其前上方按压，使其复位（图26）。本法适用于胸4以下节段椎骨错位。

7. Pressing-reduction upon the spinous process of the thoracic vertebrae with palm rim

The patient lies in prone position. The physician contacts the low rim of the suffered spinous process with the ulnar side of the hand and puts the other hand heel over his hand back. Then asks the patient to take deep breath. When patient breathes regularly and his chest wall is expanded at the end of the inhalations period, the

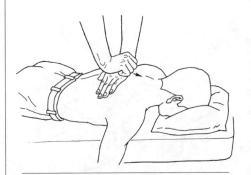

图26 胸椎棘突下掌缘按压复位法
Fig. 26 Pressing-reduction upon the spinous process of the thoracic vertebrae with palm rim

physician thrusts the spinous process directed anteriosuperiorly with the pattern of delivering force from the elbow to make resetting (Fig. 26). This manipulation is adapted to the reduction of thoracic vertebrae subluxation below the T4.

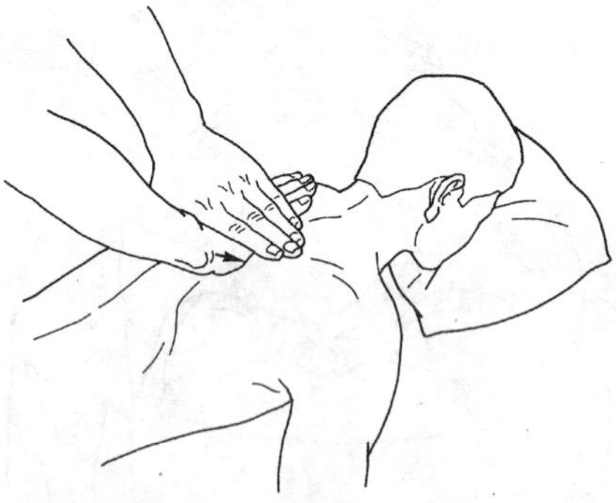

8. 肋椎关节按压复位法

患者体位同上。操作者以两手掌根重叠，按压于肋骨角；然后嘱患者深呼吸，待呼吸协调后，乘其呼气末期，呼吸肌和肋椎关节囊松弛时，适时用肘关节发力，将肋骨向其外上方按压，使其复位(图27)。本法适用于所有肋椎关节错位。

8. Pressing-reduction of the costovertebral joint

The patient lies in prone position. The physician presses the costovertebral angle with two overlapped hands. Then asks the patient to take deep breath. After the patient's breath is regular and the muscles and the capsule of the costovertebral joint is relaxed at the end of the exhalation period, the physician thrusts the rib directed laterosuperiorly to make resetting (Fig. 27). This manipulation is adapted to the reduction of costovertebral joints subluxation.

9. 骶髂关节按压松动法

患者俯卧。操作者站于其健侧，以一手掌根按住髂后上棘向患者前外方用力，另一手掌根抵住骶骨下端向患者前上方用力；嘱患者咳嗽，待其咳嗽咳出，肌肉松弛时，适时以肩臂发力，作一突发有控制推压，使骶髂关节面两侧互相错移扭转而得以松解(图28)。本法适用于骶髂关节错位而髂后上棘后凸者。此外，复位时还可在患者大腿下面垫一枕头，使髋关节后伸而利用股直肌紧张的杠杆力，协助松动(图29)。若患者髂后上棘凹陷，则医生按压的部位及用力方向均要相应改变，一手掌根按住骶骨上端向患者前下方用力，另一手掌根按压坐骨结节内侧向患者前外上方用力，使骶髂关节向相反方向扭错，即能松动(图30)。

9. Pressing-mobilization of the sacroiliac joint

The patient lies in prone position. With standing on the healthy side, the physician contacts the posterior superior sacroiliac spine to press directed anterolateroinferiorly with one palm heel, and the lower sacrum end to press directed anterior rostrally with the other palm heel.

图27 肋椎关节按压复位法
Fig. 27 Pressing-reduction of the costovertebral joint

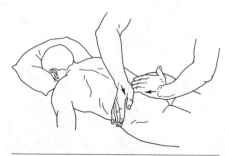

图28 骶髂关节按压松动法
Fig. 28 Pressing-mobilization of the sacroiliac joint (with projected PSIS)

Then asks the patient to make cough. When the patient's muscles is relaxed just on coughing, the physician makes a sudden and controlled thrust to cause the two facets of the sacroiliac joint to be shifted and mobilized (Fig. 28). The manipulation is adapted to the sacroiliac subluxation with the posterior superior iliac spine in posterior projection. Besides, when the manipulation is being done, the physician may also put a pillow under the suffered thigh to make the hip joint extended so as to take the advantage of the lever force produced by the strained rectus femoris, which is good for the application of the above manipulation (Fig.29). If the posterior superior iliac spine is hollow, the contact point and the direction of delivering force must be changed as follows. The physician puts one palm heels on the upper end of the sacrum and presses it anterocaudally, the other on the medial side of ischia tuberosity and thrusts it anterolaterorostrally so as to cause the two facets of the sacroiliac joint to be turned oppositely. In this way, the joint is mobilized (Fig. 30).

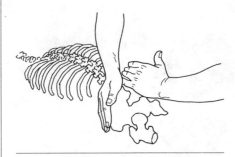

图29 骶髂关节按压松动法用力示意图

Fig. 29 Sketch graph of pressing mobilization of the sacroiliac joint (with projected PSIS)

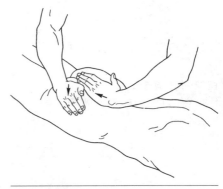

图30 骶髂关节按压松动法

Fig. 30 Pressing-mobilization of the sacroiliac joint

第二节 推擦类手法

SECTION 2 CATEGORY OF LINEAR-MOVING MANIPULATIONS

所谓推擦类手法是指操作者以指、掌或身体其他部位置于患者体表，在保持一定垂直压力下，作直线或弧线运动的一类手法(图31)。

Manipulations of linear-moving category are referred to those actions in which the manipulator puts his fingers, palm or other body parts on patient's body surface and moves straightly or cursively while keeping in constant pressing force (Fig. 31).

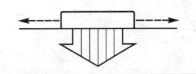

图31 推擦类手法模式图

Fig. 31 Model of category of linear-moving manipulations

一、代表手法 推法
Principal Techniques of Linear-moving Manipulations: Pushing

1. 拇指直推法

手指伸直，拇指在后，以桡侧缘触及皮肤，位于所推穴位的起点；四指在前，指尖触及所推穴位的终点；然后虎口快速一合一张，用拇指作单方向轻快推动(图32)。频率为每分钟200～240次。

1. Linear-pushing with the thumb

The physician stretches all fingers, with the thumb being put behind and the rest four fingers in front of the acting point. Then through nimble moving, in which the thumb and the other fingers are gathered and separated, the thumb is pushed forward along the point path and returned over the point path with the frequency of 200 to 240 times per minute.

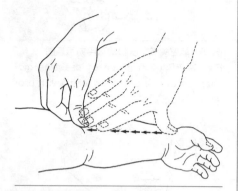

图32 拇指直推法
Fig. 32 Linear-pushing with the thumb

2. 剑指直推法

示指、中指伸直成剑指状，以罗纹面轻触皮肤，然后前臂快速摆动，带动手指轻快地作单方向推动(图33)。频率为每分钟200～240次。直推法是压力最轻的推法，要求操作时皮肤不变形，操作后皮肤不发红。推时需蘸姜汁或清水，保持皮肤湿润。直推法用于小儿推拿操作，如"推三关"、"退六腑"等，其作用根据所推穴位及方向而决定。

2. Linear-pushing with the "sword-fingers"

With the index and the middle fingers being stretched to form "sword-fingers," the physician touches the patient's skin with print regions of the two fingers, and moves the forearm forth and back quickly so as to cause the fingers to skate forward on the skin nimbly and then return back. The frequency of manipulation is 200 to 240 times a minute.

Linear-pushing is the lightest manipulation in pushing. It is required that the patient's skin be not changed in form during manipulation and in color after manipulation. When the pushing is being done, it is necessary to have the fingers a soak of clear water or ginger sauce to keep

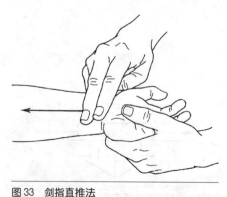

图33 剑指直推法
Fig. 33 Linear-pushing with the "sword-fingers"

the skin in moist condition. Linear-pushing is employed in pediatric Tuina such as "pushing Sanguan", "Retreating Liufu" etc. Their effects rely on both which point is acted and what direction is moved along.

3. 拇指平推法

以拇指面着力于体表,其余四指分开助力,然后用肘关节屈伸,带动拇指沿经络循行或肌纤维方向作单方向沉缓推进,连续操作5~15次。本法较直推法压力重, 适用于肩背、胸腹、腰臀及四肢操作,有疏通经络,行气活血,理筋止痛等作用,常用于治疗肩背疼痛、胸闷腹胀、痉挛拘急、关节不利等病证的治疗(图34)。

3. Flat-pushing with the thumb

The physician contacts the patient's body with the print region of the thumb that is strengthened and supported by the rest opened finger. Then drives the thumb to push forward slowly and steadily along muscles or channels and then return back by the means of extending and flexing of elbow. The manipulation is repeated 5 to 15 times. The press force of flat pushing is heavier than that of the linear pushing. It is suitable for manipulation on shoulder, back, chest, abdomen, lumbar, buttock and limb. Those such as dredging blocked channel, vivifying Qi and blood, setting tendon in order, relieving pain are its common functions. It is often applied to cure shoulder and back pain, stuffed thorax and abdomen, muscle spasm, inflexible joint and so on (Fig. 34).

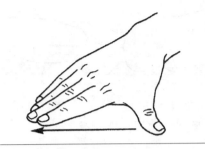

图34 拇指平推法
Fig. 34 Flat-Pushing with the thumb

4. 掌平推法

以掌根部着力于体表,手指伸直;然后用肘关节屈伸运动,带动掌面沿经络循行路线作单方向沉缓推进,连续操作5~10次(图35)。本法较拇指平推法刺激缓和,适用于腰背、胸腹、大腿等平坦部位操作,具有较好的活血解痉,宽胸理气作用,常用以治疗腰背酸痛、胸腹胀闷等病证。

4. Flat-pushing with the palm

The physician contacts the patient's body with his palm heel, with his fingers being stretched. Then drives the palm to push forward slowly and steadily along channel route by the means of extension and flexion movement of the elbow. The manipulation is repeated 5

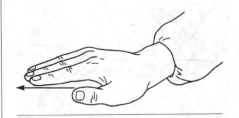

图35 掌平推法
Fig. 35 Flat-pushing with the palm

to 15 times (Fig.35). This pushing is gentler than the flat pushing with thumb. It is adapted to manipulation on those flat body regions such as back, chest, abdomen and thigh. Experts think of those effects that such as promoting blood circulation, relieving spasm, comforting thorax, regularizing Qi are good. It is usually used to heal back pain and stuffed thorax and abdomen.

5. 刨推法

用一手轻握患肢，然后以肘关节屈伸运动带动手掌沿肢体纵轴作单方向推动，连续操作5～10次。本法刺激缓和，适用于四肢操作，有舒筋活血，消肿止痛的作用，常用以四肢软组织损伤，关节痹痛的治疗(图36)。

5. Planing-pushing

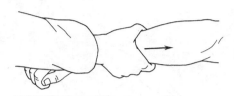

图36 刨推法
Fig. 36 Planing-pushing

The physician holds the patient's limb gently with one hand. Then drives the palm to push forward along the longitudinal axis of the limb by the means of extension and flexion of the elbow. This manipulation is repeated 5 to 10 times. The stimulation of planing-pushing is gentle and suitable for manipulation on the limbs. It has those functions, such as relaxing muscle and sinew, promoting blood circulation, lysing swollen and relieving pain. It is usually used to treat soft tissue injuries of limbs, arthritis and arthralgia (Fig. 36).

6. 拳平推法

握拳，以示指、中指、无名指、小指四指的指间关节突起处着力于体表，向一定方向推动，连续操作5～10次(图37)。本法刺激强烈，适用于肩、背、臀、腿肌肉厚实处操作，对陈伤及风湿痹痛而又感觉迟钝者，较为适用。

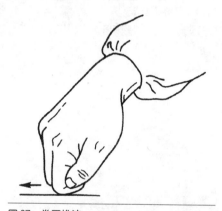

图37 拳平推法
Fig. 37 Flat-pushing with the fist

6. Flat-pushing with the fist

The physician contacts the patient's body with a fist bone bulges of the proximal interphalangeal joints of the fingers. Then drives the fist to push forward and then return back by the means of extension and flexion of the elbow. The manipulation is repeated for 5 to 10 times. This manipulation is stronger and sharp in stimulation, so it is only adapted to act on those regions where the muscles are thick and well developed such as the shoulder, the back, the buttock and the thigh. It is suitable for

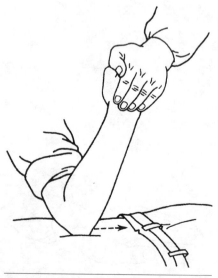

图38 肘平推法
Fig. 38 Flat-pushing with the elbow

those patients who suffered from persistent trauma, rheumatalgia and show stupid senses (Fig. 37).

7. 肘平推法
屈肘，以鹰嘴突着力于体表，向一定方向推动，连续操作5～10次(图38)。本法在推法中刺激最强，仅对身体壮实者使用。适用范围同拳平推法。

7. Flat-pushing with the elbow
The physician contacts the patient's body with a flexed elbow, then drives the elbow to push forward and return back by the means of extension and flexion of the shoulder. The manipulation is repeated 5 to 10 times. Its stimulation is the strongest in all pushing, so it is only used to those who have very strong physiques. The adapted range is like the flat-pushing with fist (Fig. 38).

8. 分推法与合推法
以两手同时操作，自肢体中轴线向两侧推动，称分推法；自肢体两侧向中轴线推动为合推法。分推法和合推法在不同部位操作有不同名称，如分(合)腕阴阳(图39)、分膻中(图40)，适合小儿推拿治疗；八字分推法适合腰背疾患治疗(图41)等。

8. Eccentric-pushing and concentric-pushing
When the two hands are manipulated simultaneously, those pushings that are moved from midline to two lateral sides are named as eccentric-pushing, while those from two lateral sides to the midline are named as concentric-pushing. The eccentric-pushing and concentric-pushing both have different names as they are applied on different parts of the body, such as Eccentrating Ying-Yang of the wrist (or concentrating Ying-Yang of the wrist)(Fig. 39), Eccentrating the Tanzhong (Fig. 40), adapted to Pediatric Tuina, "八" shaped eccentric-pushing (Fig. 41), adapted to back pain etc.

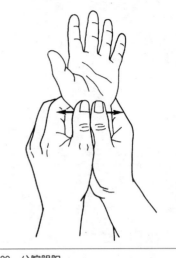

图39 分腕阴阳

Fig. 39 Eccentrating Ying-Yang of the wrist

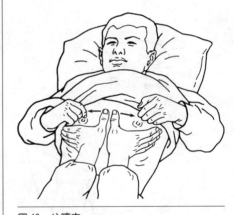

图40 分膻中

Fig. 40 Eccentrating the Tanzhong

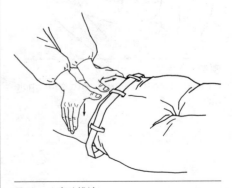

图41 八字分推法

Fig. 41 "八" shaped eccentric-pushing

二、推法的衍化
Evolution of Pushing

1. 擦法

推法的用意是推动气血在经脉中运行,故推法是单方向的推动。擦法的用意是使手掌与皮肤间及组织各层间的相互摩擦转化为热能,故擦法须往返操作。擦法的压力不能过大,以摩擦时皮肤不起皱叠为宜;擦法的移动速度较平推法快,一般掌握在每分钟100~120次。

1. Linear-rubbing

The aim of pushing is to promote Qi and blood circulation in channels and vessels. So the pushing is one way forcible moving. The goal of linear-rubbing is to transform the friction produced between the palm and the skin as well as the superficial and the deep tissues into heat energy. So the linear-rubbing must move forcibly forth and back. The press force of the linear-rubbing can't be too strong. It is suitable that no wrinkles appear on skin when the linear-rubbing is being done. The moving velocity of linear-rubbing is quicker than that of flat pushing and the frequency is about 100 to 120 times per minute.

(1)掌擦法:类似掌平推法,但压力较平推法轻,作直线往返摩擦,以深部透热为度(图42)。本法适用于肩背、胸腹等平坦部位的操作,有温经通络、宽胸理气、调理脾胃、强壮身体的作用,常用于呼吸系统疾患、消化系统疾患及体质虚弱者的治疗。

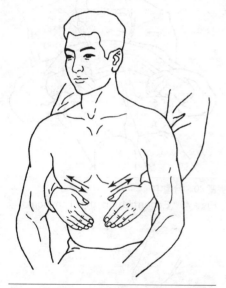

图42 掌擦法

Fig. 42 Linear-rubbing with the whole palm

(1)linear-rubbing with the whole palm: It is similar to flat pushing with palm, but its pressing force is slighter than that of the latter. The manipulator contacts the selected areas of the patient's body with the whole palm. Then drives the palm to rub the skin forth and back straightly until heat penetrates into deep tissues (Fig. 42). This manipulation is adapted to manipulation on shoulder, back, chest and abdomen. Those effects such as warming channels, dredging vessels, comforting thorax, settling Qi disorder, regulating digestive function and building up health are distinguishing. It is often employed in treating the illnesses of respiratory system and digestive system as well as poor health condition.

(2)鱼际擦法：掌指并拢微屈成虚掌，以大鱼际及掌根紧贴皮肤，作直线往返摩擦，透热为度(图43)。本法在四肢部操作较为平稳，有活血通经、消肿止痛作用，常用于四肢软组织损伤，关节肿胀及顽固性风湿痹痛的治疗。

(2)linear-rubbing with the thenar eminence: The manipulator closes and slightly flexes all fingers to make a vacuous palm, and puts the thenar eminence and the heel of the palm on skin. Then drives the hand to rub forth and back straightly until heat penetrates into the deep tissues of the manipulated area(Fig. 43).This manipulation is more steadily in manipulated on limbs.It has functions such as promoting blood circulation, dredging blocked channels and vessels, lysising swollen and relieving pain etc.Those troubles such as injuries of the soft tissues on limbs,swollen joints and persistent rheumatagia are all adapted.

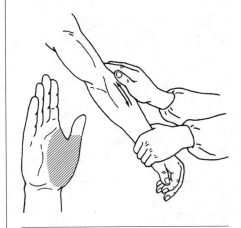

图43 鱼际擦法

Fig. 43 Linear-rubbing with the thenar eminence

(3)侧擦法：掌指伸直，以手掌小鱼际部位紧贴皮肤，作直线往返摩擦(图44)。本法温热作用较强，适用于腰背、骶部、小腹等处操作，有温经散寒、补肾强身、活血祛风作用，常用于治疗腰背疼痛、筋脉拘急、小腹冷痛、体质虚弱等。擦法操作时，可在局部涂少许润滑剂，既可保护皮肤，又可使热量深透。擦法使用后，皮肤可能轻度损伤，故擦法多在其他手法之后应用。不可在擦法之后再在局部应用其他手法，以免破皮。

(3)Linear-rubbing with hypothenar: The manipulator contacts patient's skin with the hypothenar side of the palm, while his fingers are stretched. Then drives the hand to rub forward and backward straightly until heat penetrates into deep tissues of the manipulated area(Fig. 44). This manipulation has strong warm effect and is adapted to manipulation on back, sacrum and lower abdominal regions.Warming channels, eliminating cold evil, reinforcing kidney, building up health, promoting blood circulation and dispelling wind evil are all its distinguished functions.It often applied to the treatments of back pain, muscle and tendon spasms, cold and pain in the lower abdomen,worse healthy condition etc. When

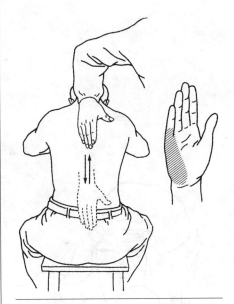

图44 侧擦法

Fig. 44 Linear-rubbing with the hypothenar

the linear-rubbing is manipulated, one should smear some grease on skin in order to protect skin as well as promote heat penetrating. After linear-rubbing, there may be slight injury on skin, therefor the linear rubbing must be used at the end of manipulations so as to avoid abrasion of skin.

2. 拨法

或称弹拨法。推法与擦法操作时，垂直按压力小而直线移动幅度大，操作者手与患者体表间产生相对摩擦。拨法操作时，垂直按压力量大而直线移动幅度小。以拇指端按在治疗部位上，作短距离直线拨动，使深层组织之间产生相互错移摩动（图45）。本法刺激强烈，有分离粘连、舒筋解痉的作用，适用于压痛点操作，治疗软组织粘连、挛缩。

2. Plucking

Also named as catapult plucking. When the pushing and linear-rubbing are being done, the pressing force is lighter while the moving range is longer, so there is friction between hand and skin. When the plucking is being done, the press force is heavier while the moving range is shorter, and the thumb fixes on the skin and moves at a very short range to make each layer of deep tissue ground relatively (Fig. 45). This manipulation stimulus is strong and it is usually applied to trigger point to treat the adherence and contraction of soft tissue. It can peel off adherence, relax muscle and sinew and relieve spasm.

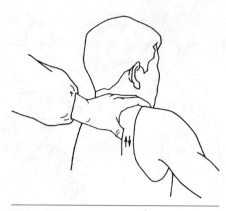

图45 拨法
Fig. 45 Plucking

3. 抹法

以拇指平推法或掌平推法在头面部按固定程序操作，称抹法（图46）。抹法操作方式是：医生面对病人站立，用双手轻扶患者头部两侧，两拇指自印堂穴交替向上抹至前额，往返15次；随后两拇指自印堂分抹至两侧太阳穴并揉太阳数次，仍合推至印堂，往返15次；再从印堂沿眼眶周围反复抹动15次；最后，从印堂沿鼻柱两侧、颧骨下缘分抹至两耳前听宫穴，并返回印堂，往返15次（图46）。以上动作要连续不断，一气呵成。术后患者顿觉眼目清亮，头脑清醒。抹头面具有祛风醒目、宁神降压的作用，常用于治疗感冒、头痛、失眠、高血压等症。

3. Wiping

Wiping is referred to those flat-pushing with the thumb or with the palm on the face and head following

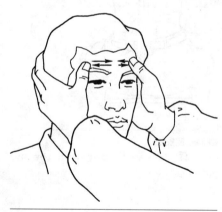

图46 抹法
Fig. 46 Wiping

a fixed program. This program is as below: The physician stands in front of the patient, with his hands being put on both side of the patient's temporal regions, and moves the thumbs in turn for 15 times by wiping from the point Yintang to the point Shenting, and then from the point Yintang to the point Taiyang, from the point Jingming to the point Taiyang along the upper and lower borders of the eyesockets and from Yintang through Jingming, the lateral sides of the nose, the low rims of the cheek bones to Tinggong. All the wiping routes are repeated for 15 times(Fig.46). The above actions must be done continuously and not be broken. After wiping, the patient immediately refreshes seeing and thinking. Because wiping on the face and head may dispel the wind evil, clear seeing, calm mind and depress higher blood pressure etc., those illnesses such as cold, headache, insomnia, hypertension show good responses to it.

4. 扫散法

医生以一手轻轻扶住患者头部，另一手指伸直，以拇指桡侧面及其余四指指端，同时贴于头颞部，稍用力在耳上后方(胆经循行部位)自前上向后下作弧形单向摩动。本法具有平肝潜阳，祛风止痛作用，常用于头痛、眩晕、高血压等证(图47)。

4. Sweeping

The doctor gently supports patient's head with his one hand and contacts the patient's temporal region with the radial side of thumb and the tips of four fingers of the other hand. Then moves the hand along an arc route from the temporal region to occipital region(along the Gall Bladder Channel route), directed anterior-superior to posterior-inferior. This manipulation possesses effects of inhibiting Liver Yang, dispelling the wind evil and relieving pain, therefore those illnesses such as headache, dizziness, hypertension show good responses to it(Fig. 47).

5. 拘法

与扫散法相似，但操作者位于患者后面操作。两拇指按在枕骨两侧，把两手其他指并拢微屈成钩状，以示指中节、末节的桡侧缘着力，从两侧太阳穴起向后沿耳上后方作弧形摩动至

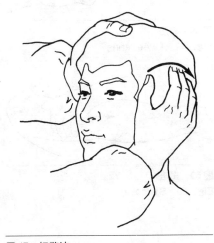

图47 扫散法
Fig. 47 Sweeping

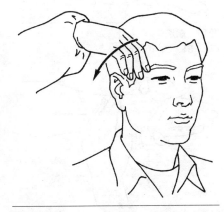

图48 拘法
Fig. 48 Canceling

枕骨两侧，反复数次(图48)。作用同扫散法。

5. Canceling

It is like the sweeping. The doctor stands behind the patient. With his two thumbs being put on the lateral sides of the occipital bone, his radial sides of the index fingers that are slightly flexed as "hook", as well as the rest fingers, are put on the temporal regions. Then drives the fingers to rub on the temporal regions along an arc route from the point Taiyang to the occipital bone.The manipulation is repeated for several times(Fig. 48).Its effects are similar to those of the sweeping.

6. 勒法

又称搊法、理法。以屈曲的中指、示指夹住指(或趾)后，向指端滑勒，各指(或趾)均勒一遍。

6. Tweezering

It is also named for stripping or arranging.The doctor clamps patient's finger between flexed index finger and middle finger, then slips out of the finger tip. Each finger(or toe) is manipulated a time(Fig.49).

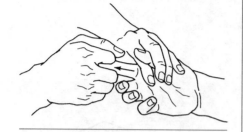

图49 勒法
Fig. 49 Tweezering

7. 捋顺法

以掌推法在四肢伸侧自近端推向远端，称捋法(图50)；四肢屈侧自远端推向近端称顺法(图51)。

7. Stripping and Conforming

When manipulated on the limbs, pushing with palm moved from the proximal to the distal on the extensional side is named as stripping(Fig. 50), while from the distal to the proximal on the flexion side is named as conforming (Fig. 51).

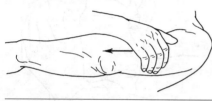

图50 捋法
Fig. 50 Stripping

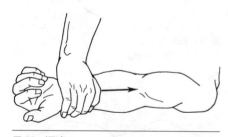

图51 顺法
Fig. 51 Conforming

8. 拂法、刮法

以四指罗纹面轻快地单方向掠擦皮肤的手法称拂法(图52)，与指直推法相近。以指罗纹面较重地单方向掠擦皮肤的手法，或以匙缘、铜钱边缘掠擦皮肤至皮下瘀血的手法，均称刮法(图53)。

8. Skimming and Scraping

The manipulation in which one take the print regions of the four fingers to skim gently on the skin is called for skimming (Fig. 52). It is very similar to the manipula-

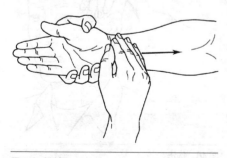

图52 拂法
Fig. 52 Skimming

tion linear pushing. If the manipulative force is heavy, it will be named as scraping. Those manipulations that rub skin with a spoon rim or a coin rim are also named as scraping (Fig. 53).

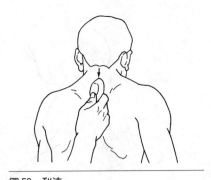

图 53 刮法
Fig. 53 Scraping "sha"

第三节　摩揉类手法
SECTION 3 CATEGORY OF CIRCULAR-MOVING MANIPULATIONS

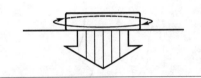

图 54 摩揉类手法模式图
Fig. 54 model of the Category of the Circular-moving manipulations

所谓摩揉类手法是指操作者以指、掌或身体其他部位接触患者体表，在保持一定垂直压力下作环旋运动的一类手法。摩揉类手法可用图 54 模拟表示。

Category of circular-moving manipulations means those actions during which the manipulator puts his fingers, palms or other parts of body on the patient's body and moves them circularly while keeping in constant pressing force. This category can be modeled by Fig. 54.

一、代表手法　摩法
Principal Techniques of Circular-moving Manipulations: Circular-rubbing

摩为抚摩之意。摩法有两种操作方式，用示、中、无名指指面抚摩称指摩法，用手掌面抚摩称掌摩法。

Rubbing means to stroke. There are two main manipulative manners in circular-rubbing. The manipulative manner in which the print regions of the index, middle and ring fingers are put on the patient's body is named as circular-rubbing with the fingers while the whole palm is put on body is named as circular-rubbing with palm.

1. 指摩法

肘关节微屈，腕关节放松，手指自然伸直，以示、中、无名指罗纹面轻轻接触患者体表，以前臂主动摆动，带动腕关节作环转运动，使操作者指面在患者体表产生环旋摩擦（图55）。

1. Circular-rubbing with the fingers

With his elbow flexed slightly, the wrist and fingers extended naturally, the manipulator puts the print regions of the fingers on the patient's body surface, then swings the forearm actively to rotate the wrist joint and cause the fingerprints to rub on the body surface passively in circular form (Fig.55).

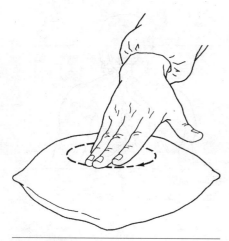

图55 指摩法
Fig. 55 Circular-rubbing with the fingers

2. 掌摩法

操作方式基本同指摩法，但操作者以掌面与患者体表接触（图56）。

2. Circular-rubbing with the palm

The manipulative pattern is similar to circular-rubbing with the fingers. But the manipulator touches patient's skin with whole palm(Fig.56).

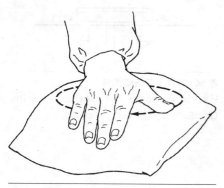

图56 掌摩法
Fig. 56 Circular-rubbing with the palm

摩法操作时，动作宜轻柔，压力不要太大，顺时针方向与逆时针方向环摩均可，每分钟操作频率为100～120次。摩法刺激舒适缓和，适用于胸腹与胁肋部操作，也可在其他部位的损伤肿痛处操作。具有宽胸理气、疏肝和中、消积导滞和活血散瘀的作用，治疗胸肋胀闷、脘腹疼痛、消化不良、泄泻便秘及外伤肿胀等证。

On applying circular-rubbings, the motion should be gentle, the force should not be too heavy, and both rubbings in clockwise and anti-clockwise are feasible. The manipulative frequency is about 100 to 120 times per minute. The stimulation of circular-rubbing is comfortable and mild. It is suitable for manipulation on the thorax, the abdomen, the rib regions as well as other parts where the soft tissues is injured and swollen. It has comforting thorax, regulating Qi, smoothing liver, regulating digestive function and promoting blood circulation etc. distinguished effects.So the circular-rubbing is used to treat stuffed thorax and rib regions, stomach and abdomen pain, indigestion, diarrhea, constipation, sprain or contusion of soft tissue.

古代应用摩法时常在施术皮肤涂以药膏，以加强手法的治疗作用，称之为膏摩。

In ancient times, the doctor often applied some herb paste on skin to enhance the curative effects of manipulation when the circular-rubbing was done. This is named as paste circular-rubbing.

二、摩法的衍化
Evolution of Circular-rubbing

1. 揉法

在摩法操作的基础上，增加向下的垂直压力，减小环旋运动的幅度，使操作者指、掌粘附于患者体表皮肤保持相对不动，而带动皮下浅层组织在深层组织界面上环转揉动，称为揉法。故《保赤推拿法》说："揉者，医以指按儿经穴，不离其处而环转之也。"《厘正按摩要术》称："揉法以手宛转回环，宜轻宜缓，绕于其上也，是从摩法生出者。"

1. Kneading

Based on the action of circular-rubbing, if the vertical press force is increased and the range of circular moving reduced, the manipulator's hand will adhere to the patient's skin and keep in relative fixed relation, but drive the shallow subcutaneous tissue to knead on the deep tissue circularly. The manipulation becomes kneading. So the ancient book, *Bao Chi Tui Na Fa* said:"The kneading is referred to the manipulation in which the doctor puts his fingers to press baby's acupoints and rotates on the skin circularly. And should not leave his fingers from the acupoints." The book *Li Zheng An Mo Yao Shu* states that,"Kneading means to revolve, to circle on the skin with hand. It should be light and mild. It is developed from the circular-rubbing."

揉法有指腹揉、掌根揉、大鱼际揉、拇指外侧揉等4种操作方式。

There are as many as four different manipulative patterns in kneading. They are kneading with the fingerprints, kneading with the palm heel, kneading with the thenar, and kneading with radial side of the thumb etc.

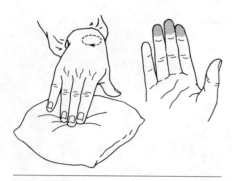

图57 指腹揉
Fig. 57 Kneading with the fingerprints

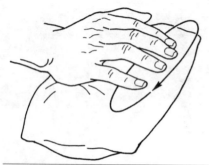

图58 掌根揉
Fig.58 Kneading with palm heel

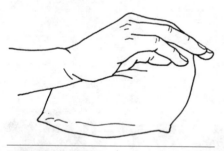

图59 大鱼际揉前视
Fig. 59 Front view of kneading with the thenar

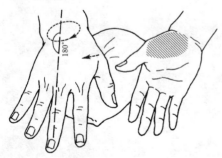

图60 大鱼际揉前摆
Fig. 60 Anterior swinging of kneading with the thenar

(1)指腹揉：以示、中、无名指指腹揉动，操作方法与指摩法相仿(图57)。

(1)kneading with the fingerprints：It is referred to kneading on patient's skin with the print regions of the index, middle and ring fingers. The manipulative manner is similar to circular-rubbing with fingers (Fig. 57).

(2)掌根揉：操作者腕关节略背屈，手指自然屈曲，以掌根部着力于患者体表作环旋揉动。操作方法与掌摩法相似(图58)。

(2)kneading with palm heel：The manipulator extends his wrist joint slightly, flexes his fingers naturally, and puts his palm heel on the patient's skin to knead circularly. The action manner is very similar to circular-rubbing with the palm (Fig. 58).

(3)大鱼际揉：肘关节屈曲120°，腕关节放松，肘腕大致在同一水平线上；手尺侧缘在前，桡侧缘在后，以手掌大鱼际部位接触患者体表(图59)；然后前臂作主动摆动，带动腕关节、第一腕掌关节环转运动，使大鱼际附着于皮肤，皮下组织在深层组织界面上环旋揉动(图60, 61)。

(3)kneading with the thenar：With the elbow joint flexed about 120°, the wrist joint relaxed, the manipulator keeps the two joints in level and the ulnar side of the hand in anterior while the radial side in posterior. Then puts the thenar eminence on the patient's skin (Fig. 59), and swings the forearm actively to drive the wrist joint and the first metacarpophalangeal joint to turn around. In this way, the thenar eminence and the skin and the subcutaneous tissues is moved together on the interface of the deep tissue(Fig. 60, 61).

(4)拇指桡侧揉：操作方式与大鱼际揉相仿,操作者以拇指桡侧缘接触患者体表揉动(图62, 63, 64)。

(4)kneading with the radial side of the thumb：The manipulative manner is similar to kneading with the thenar. But the manipulator touches patient's skin with his radial side of the thumb to knead (Fig. 62,63,64).

揉法操作宜轻快柔和，压力不可过大，摆动频率为每分钟

120～160次。

The kneading manipulation should be slight, quick and gentle, but not be heavy. Its frequency is about 120 to 160 times per minute.

揉法刺激轻柔缓和,其适用范围较广。指腹揉多用于小儿推拿,掌揉法常用于脘腹、胁肋腰背等大面积平坦部位的操作,大鱼际揉适用于头面部、胸胁部操作,拇指外侧揉适用于眼眶周围、肋间隙操作。具有宽胸理气、健脾和胃、活血化瘀、舒筋解痉、消肿定痛的作用,治疗胸闷胁痛、脘腹胀满、泄泻便秘、头痛眩晕、神衰失眠、口眼㖞斜、外伤肿痛等证。

The stimulation of kneading is gentle and mild. Its adapting range is very broad. The kneading with finger prints is applied to pediatric Tuina. The kneading with palm heel is often used for manipulating on those body parts whose surfaces are flat, such as abdomen, rib region and back. The kneading with thenar is frequently employed for manipulation on head, face, thorax and rib regions. And the kneading with radial side of thumb is used for manipulating on eyehole and intercostal space. The manipulation have those effects such as conforming thorax, regularizing Qi, tonifying the spleen and attempting the stomach, promoting blood circulation to eliminate homeostasis, relaxing muscles and tendons, removing swollen and relieving pain etc. Those illness such as thoracic and hypochondriac pain, fullness in stomach and abdomen, diarrhea, constipation, headache, dizziness, insomnia due to neurasthenia, facial paralysis, injury of soft tissues etc. are all its indications.

2. 运法

在指摩法的基础上,减轻向下的压力,使拇指或中指端轻触小儿穴位皮肤,然后作缓慢的环旋摩擦运动,称运法(图65)。运法操作时,患者皮肤不变形,仅引起触觉;而摩按操作时,皮肤轻微凹陷、变形、有压觉。有时小儿推拿中把压力很轻的弧形推动,亦称为运法。运法宜轻不易重,宜缓不宜急,每分钟操作60～80次。运法适用于小儿手上穴位操作,如运八卦、运水入土等,其治疗作用根据穴位而定。

2. Transporting

Based on the action of circular-rubbing, if the press-

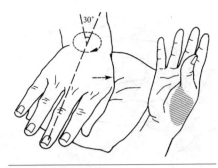

图61 大鱼际揉后摆

Fig. 61 Posterior swinging of kneading with the thenar

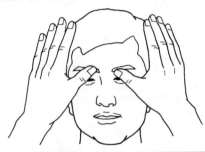

图62 拇指桡侧揉

Fig. 62 Kneading with the radial side of the thumb

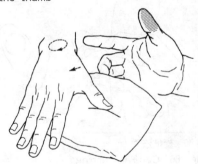

图63 拇指桡侧揉前摆

Fig. 63 Anterior swinging of kneading with the radial side of the thumb

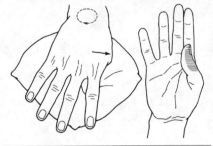

图64 拇指桡侧揉后摆

Fig. 64 Posterior swinging of kneading with the radial side of the thumb

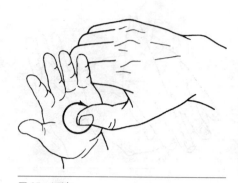

图 65 运法
Fig. 65 Transporting

ing force is decreased, the tip of the thumb or the middle finger are gently touched the skin of baby, and the rubbing is moved very slowly, the manipulation is changed transporting(Fig.65). During transporting manipulation, the baby's skin is not out of shape and only the tactile sensation is felled.But during circular-rubbing, the skin is slightly depressed and the pressures sensation is caused.Sometimes the arch shaped pushing whose force is very light is also called as transporting in pediatric Tuina.Transporting should be slight and mild, but not heavy and rapid.It should be manipulated 60 to 80 times per minute. Transporting is adapted to manipulating on the acupoints of baby's hand, such as transporting Eight Diagrams, transporting Water to Earth. The curative effects are determined by what points are acted.

3. 旋推法

在运法的基础上,略增加压力,减小环转运动幅度,加快操作频率,则称为旋推法(图66)。旋推法适用于小儿推拿指端穴位操作,操作频率为每分钟200～240次,其治疗作用偏于补。

3. Circular-pushing

Based on the action of transporting, if the pressing force is increased and the range of circular moving is reduced, the manipulation is called as circular-pushing (Fig. 66). Circular pushing is suitable for acting on the acupoints on baby's fingers. The frequency is 200 to 240 times per minute. Its curative effects are inclined to tonifying.

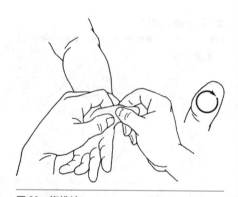

图 66 旋推法
Fig. 66 Circular-pushing

三、复合手法　按揉法
Compound Manipulation: Pressing-Kneading

在按法的基础上增加缓慢的环转揉动；或在揉法的基础上,增加向下按压的力量,为按揉法(图67)。按揉法增加了对穴位的刺激性,但不增加患者疼痛程度,适用于穴位操作。

Based on the pressing manipulation and adding slow circular motion, or based on the kneading manipulation and increasing the pressing force, the manipulation becomes pressing-kneading(Fig. 67).The pressing-kneading increase stimulation to the acupoints, but doesn't raise pain level.It is suitable for manipulation on acupoints.

[附] 摩揉法的操作练习
[Appendix] Manipulation Exercise of Circular-rubbing and Kneading

　　初学推拿手法者，在作摩法、揉法练习时，常觉动作生硬欠灵活。究其原因，一是未找到正确的操作方式，二是腕关节缺乏柔韧性。建议学习者作以下练习动作：①两手十指交叉，然后作腕部扭转动作。每次练习1~2分钟，以增加腕关节柔韧性(图68)。②腕关节放松，然后以前臂摆动，带动腕关节作侧向摆腕动作(图69)。这种侧向摆腕的前臂运动方式，就是摩揉法的前臂运动方式。只不过侧向摆腕时，手是游离的，其运动幅度大于腕部；当摩揉法操作指掌粘附于某一点后，腕部形成运动中心，自然就协调地摆动起来了。仔细体会一下侧向摆腕的前臂运动方式，然后按这一运动方式练习摩、揉法。将很快能掌握其操作方式。

　　When one drills circular rubbing or kneading, the beginner will often feel the action being stiff and rough. What is the matter? The first, one has not found out the right manipulative manner.The second, his wrist joint lacks pliability and toughness.It is suggested that the learner follows the below drills：① Turning the wrist roundly with crossing the ten fingers for 1 to 2 minutes each time to increase the pliability and toughness of the wrist joint(Fig.68). ② With relaxing of the wrist joint, swinging the forearm actively to make the wrist joint swung from side to side(Fig.69), in which the motion manner of the forearm is just the motion manners of the circular-rubbing and the kneading on doing the exercise, the hand is free and its motion range is broader than that of the wrist. While during circular-rubbing and kneading, since the hand is adhered to a point, the wrist becomes motion center and swings naturally and coordinately. Considering how the forearm acts during swinging wrist side to side, then drilling circular-rubbing and kneading according to this manner, one will quickly familiarize the

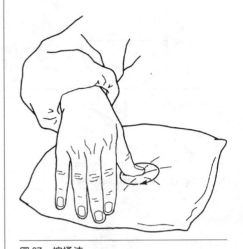

图67　按揉法
Fig. 67　Pressing-kneading

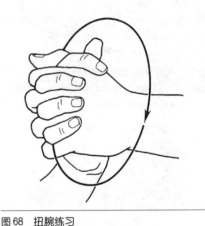

图68　扭腕练习
Fig. 68　Exercise of turning wrists around

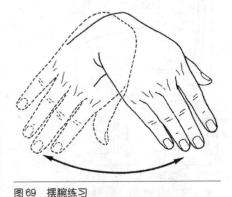

图69　摆腕练习
Fig. 69　Exercise of swinging wrist

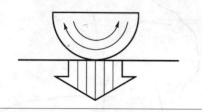

图70 推拿类手法模式图
Fig. 70 Model of the Category of the Pushing-rolling manipulations

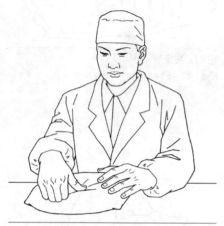

图71 一指禅推法姿势（前视）
Fig. 71 Posture of Dhyana-thumb-pushing(Frontal view)

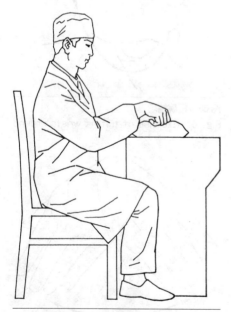

图72 一指禅推法姿势（侧视）
Fig. 72 Posture of Dhyana-thumb-pushing(Lateral view)

right manipulative manner.

第四节 推拿类手法
SECTION 4 CATEGORY OF PUSHING-ROLLING MANIPULATIONS

所谓推拿类手法，是指以操作者的指端、手背与患者体表形成曲面接触，然后前臂主动摆动，带动腕关节(或拇指小关节)作屈伸运动，使接触部位来回滚动的一类操作。推拿类手法是中医推拿手法的特色和精华。推拿类手法可用图70模拟表示。

Category of pushing-rolling manipulation refers to those actions during which the manipulator makes his finger tip or hand back camber shapes to touch the patient's body surface, then his forearm swings actively to drive the wrist joint(or joints of thumb) to extend and flex and makes the contact part roll forward and backward. These manipulations are the characters and the creams of the Tuina of TCM. Fig. 70 can modify them.

一、代表手法1 一指禅推法
Principal Techniques 1 of Pushing-Rolling Manipulations: Dhyana-Thumb-Pushing

练习一指禅推法前，必须摆正姿势。端坐，含胸拔背；肩关节放松，肩胛骨自然下垂；上臂肌肉放松，肘部屈曲下垂，略低于腕部；腕关节放松，垂屈；四指自然屈曲，握成虚拳；拇指伸直，指端自然着力于一点，指掌侧遮盖拳眼，指间关节纹正好与示指桡则缘相贴(图71，72，73)。

Before drilling the Dhyana-thumb-pushing, it is necessary to rectify posture as followed.The manipulator sits uprightly with the thoracic and lumbar spine being flexed slightly, the shoulder and the arm relaxed, the scapula bone descended naturally, the elbow flexed and descended lower than the wrist, the wrist flexed fully, and the fingers flexed naturally to make a empty fist. Then puts the thumb tip, which is extended naturally, on a point. Thus the palm side of the thumb is just covered the "fist eye" and its transverse crease of the interphalangeal joint kept close to index finger(Fig.71, 72, 73).

然后，操作者自我检查一下上肢除腕关节外，是否已经完全放松(初学者腕关节处可能有紧张感)。如感到某处僵硬不舒服，应随时调整之。只有在完全放松的基础上，才能做到动作灵活，操作持久，蓄力于掌，发力于指，刚柔相济，力透溪谷。否则，可能把动作练僵而不易纠正。

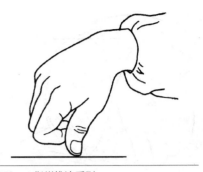

图73 一指禅推法手形
Fig. 73 Hand shape of Dhyana-thumb-pushing

Then, the manipulator checks himself if the upper limb is completely relaxed except the wrist(The learner probably has the tight feeling on the wrist region). If somewhere is felt stiff and uncomfortable, one must correct it at any time. Only based on complete relax, will one be possible to achieve moving nimbly, manipulating durably, delivering force from the palm to the thumb, combine forceful and gentle, penetrating into muscles and tendons. Otherwise, the action will become rigid probably and hardly corrected it again.

上肢完全放松后，再练习动作。先将肘关节略伸，前臂前摆旋后，腕部前移，带动拇指外展、伸直，虎口张开，以罗纹面接触米袋(图74)；随后，肘关节略屈，前臂回摆旋前，腕部后移，带动拇指内收、屈曲(也可不屈曲)，以指端近指甲处接触米袋(图75)。把上述动作连续起来操作，不使有瞬间停顿，就成为一指禅推法操作。操作中还应注意，前摆时前臂尺侧低于桡侧，回摆至极限时，前臂背面持平(图76)。

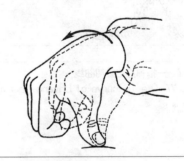

图74 一指禅推法前摆
Fig. 74 Forward swinging of Dhyana-thumb-pushing

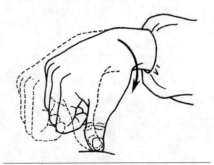

图75 一指禅推法回摆
Fig. 75 Back swinging of Dhyana-thumb-pushing

After the upper limb is completely relaxed, one can drill the manipulation. At first, the elbow joint is extended slightly, the forearm is supinated and swung forward, and the wrist region moved forward. Thus the thumb is driven to abduct and straight, the first web of the hand is opened, and the thumb print is touched the exercise bag(Fig. 74). Then, the elbow joint is flexed slightly, the forearm pronated and swung backward, and the wrist moved backward. In this way, the thumb is driven to abduct and flex (It is also allowed not to

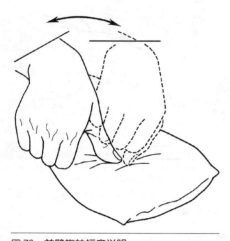

图 76 前臂旋转幅度说明
Fig. 76 Illustration of the forearm rotation

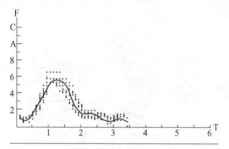

图 77 一指禅推法叠加曲线
Fig. 77 Pile-up curve of Dhyana-thumb-pushing

flex), the first web is closed, and the thumb tip is touched the exercise bag(Fig. 75). With linking these actions, the right manipulative manner of dhyana-thumb-pushing is get. It should be noted that, the ulnar side of the forearm is lower than the radial side during the forward swinging, but at the same level when the wrist swings backward to its limit(Fig. 76).

一指禅推法操作时，要求动作协调灵活，压力均匀柔和，不可时轻时重，时快时慢。图77为典型一指禅推法的压力曲线，注意其峰值、波形、波宽的一致性。一指禅推法初练时，要求拇指端吸定于一点，不能随着前后摆动而滑移。然后在吸定的基础上，再练习拇指沿一定路线移动的控制能力，要求其在操作过程中，能使指端随心所欲地沿着一定的路线(通常为经络路线)往返移动，做到紧推慢移。此外，操作时拇指端不可有意识向下按压，操作频率为每分钟140～160次。

The manipulation of the dhyana-thumb-pushing is required that the action be harmonious and nimble, the press force be uniform and gentle. Sometimes light and sometimes heavy as well as sometimes quick and sometimes slow are both not allowed. The Fig. 77 is a typical dynamic curve of the dhyana-thumb-pushing. Pay attention on that its peak values, wave shapes and wave width are all very similar. When you start drilling the manipulation, you ought to keep the thumb tip on one point, but not make it slide during swinging of the wrist and the forearm. When you control the above requirements, you can learn to control your thumb tip along some specially selected lines(usually a channel route) to and fro. Followed your inclinations during manipulation. Besides, it is not permitted to press down deliberately and over forcefully. Its frequency is about 140 to 160 times per minute.

一指禅推法接触面小而柔软，对经络穴位发挥持续不断、柔和有力的刺激，适用于全身穴位、经络路线的操作。有疏筋通络、行气活血、调节内脏功能的作用，尤适宜于内、妇、儿科疾病的治疗，对头痛、失眠、口眼㖞斜、泄泻、便秘、月经不调有较好的治疗作用。

The contact area of the dhyana-thumb-pushing is

small and soft. It can stimulate the channels and acupoints continuously, gently and forcefully. All the acupoints and the channel routes are adapted to be acted by this manipulation. It can relax muscles and tendons, dredge blocked channels and collaterals, promote Qi and blood circulation, adjust the functions of viscera. It is especially suitable for treating the diseases of internal medicine, gynecology and pediatrics. Those illnesses such as headache, insomnia, facial paralysis, diarrhea, constipation and irregular menstruation show good responses to this manipulation.

二、一指禅推法的衍化
Evolution of Dhyana-Thumb-Pushing

由于人体各部位结构的不同，一指禅推法的这种标准操作方式在人体实际操作中，有时会感到困难。因此一指禅推拿流派在实际操作中，根据人体各部位结构的特点，创造了许多变法。常用的有：

The above mentioned standard manipulative manner of dhyana-thumb-pushing sometimes is difficult to do in clinic due to the construction differences in different parts of the human body surface. So the Dhyana-thumb-pushing school of Tuina has created several variations. The frequently used are the followed:

1. 偏峰推

在头面、胸肋部操作时，垂腕握拳方式可能造成手指与体表的撞击。故一指禅推法在头面部操作时，腕关节略屈曲，手指伸直，以拇指偏峰处着力于一定部位，作前后推动(图78)。实际上偏峰推的操作方式已与拇指桡侧揉法相近。头面部偏峰推的移动路线是有规律的。

1. Thumb-pushing with the side tip

When the standard manipulative manner is applied on the head, face or thorax regions, the manner in which the manipulator flexes his wrist and holds his fist may make the fingers bump against the body surface. So if manipulating on these regions with Dhyana-thumb-pushing, one should flex the wrist joint slightly, extend

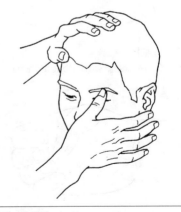

图78 偏峰推
Fig. 78 Thumb-pushing with the side tip

the fingers and put the radial side tip of the thumb on a point to swing forward and backward(Fig. 78). In fact, this manipulative manner and the kneading with the radial side of thumb are fairly alike. The moving route of thumb pushing with side tip on head and face is fixed.

2. 蝴蝶双飞

风池为推拿治疗要穴。临床上以一指禅推法刺激风池穴时，通常以双手拇指操作，形象地称为蝴蝶双飞(图79)。

2. Couple flying butterflies

Fengchi is an important acupoint in clinic of Tuina therapy. General, if manipulated on neck, one should usually use two hands to do thumb-pushing with tips so as to stimulate the bilateral acupoints Fengchi at same time. Therefore, it is vividly named as couple flying butterflies(Fig. 79)

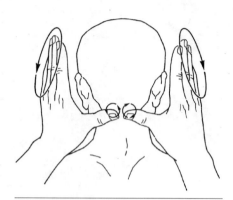

图79 蝴蝶双飞
Fig. 79 Couple flying butterflies

3. 屈指推

一指禅推法在项部操作时，不容易吸定；另外，颈椎病患者项肌强硬，压力较轻时，力量难以深透。将拇指屈曲，以拇指指间关节与指甲盖为着力面作一指禅推，称为屈指推(图80，81)。屈指推压力大，刺激强，吸定性好，适合于项枕部、关节骨缝处操作。

3. Pushing with flexed thumb

It is not easy to keep the thumb tip at a point when the dhyana-thumb-pushing is done on the nape region. Moreover, since the nape muscles of the cervical spondylopathy sufferers are rigid, the manipulation force is hardly to penetrate into the deep tissues. The manipulative manner that the back side of the interphalangeal joint of flexed thumb is taken for touch area to do dhyana-thumb-pushing is referred as pushing with flexed thumb (Fig. 80, 81). Its pressure is higher, its stimulation is stronger, and its stability is better. So the pushing with flexed thumb is adapted to manipulation on the nape-occipital region and the interval of bones and joins.

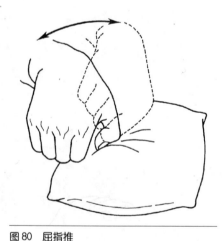

图80 屈指推
Fig. 80 Pushing with flexed thumb

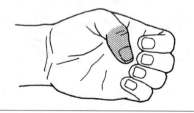

图81 屈指推接触面
Fig. 81 Touch aspect of pushing with flexed thumb

4. 双手交叉扶持推

四指伸直，虎口张开，以双手拇指指腹着力于患者颈椎对侧缘，四指则扶持于颈外侧，稳定操作，然后双手一起摆动，沿颈椎两侧推移。该法稳定性好，工作效率也高(图82)。

4. Dhyana-thumb-pushing supported by the crossed hands

With extended fingers and opened first web, the manipulator puts two crossed thumbs on the two opposite sides of the patient's cervical spine and the rest fingers on the homolateral sides of the neck to stabilize the hands. Then swings two hands and moves the thumbs along the cervical spine in the meantime. The manipulation has a good stability and a high efficiency (Fig. 82).

5. 单手扶持推

在四肢关节处操作时，一般用单手扶持推(图83)。

5. Thumb-pushing supported by single hand

Manipulated on the joints of limbs, generally used manner is the thumb-pushing supported by single hand (Fig. 83).

6. 推摩法

本法是一指禅推法和摩法的复合操作，以拇指吸定于某穴，余四指指腹在另外腹壁处作环旋摩动。推摩法适用于腹部操作(图84)。

6. Dhyana-thumb-pushing and Circular-rubbing

This manipulation is the compound manipulation combined the dhyana-thumb-pushing with the circular-rubbing. The manipulator keeps the thumb at acupoints and makes the rest fingers rub on the abdomen wall circularly. The dhyana-thumb-pushing and circular-rubbing is suitable for abdomen region(Fig. 84).

7. 缠法

加快一指禅推法操作频率，使之超过每分钟200次以上，则称为缠法。缠法一般以偏峰着力，前后摆动的幅度亦较小，波动缓和而频率高。缠法适用于外科疮疡初起及外伤肿痛处操作，有较好的消散作用。

7. Twining

If the manipulative frequency of dhyana-thumb-pushing is over 200 times per minute, it is named as twining. Generally, the twining is required that the manipulator touches body with the radial side tip of the thumb and

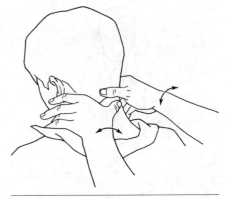

图82 双手交叉扶持推
Fig. 82 Dhyana-thumb-pushing supported by the crossed hands

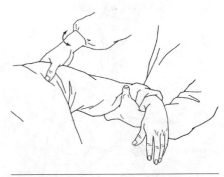

图83 单手扶持推
Fig. 83 Dhyana-thumb-pushing supported by single hand

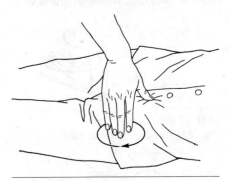

图84 推摩法
Fig. 84 Dhyana-thumb-pushing and circular-rubbing

swings in minor range, mitigative wave and high frequency. The twining is suitable on the local regions where a boil or furuncle in initiate stage or the injury with swollen and pain. It has a good dispersing effect.

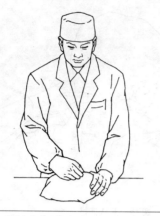

图85 㨰法姿势（前视）
Fig. 85 Posture of rolling (Frontal view)

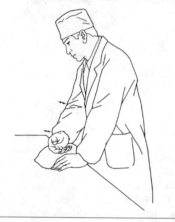

图86 㨰法姿势（侧视）
Fig. 86 Posture of rolling (lateral view)

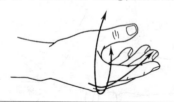

图87 手背弧面
Fig. 87 Camber of hand back

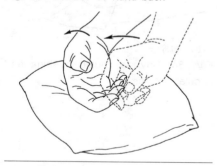

图88 㨰法前滚运动
Fig. 88 Anterior roll of rolling

三、代表手法2　㨰法
Principal Techniques 2 of Pushing-Rolling Manipulation: Rolling

㨰法操作练习前，应摆正姿势。操作者站立，两脚略前后分开，上身前倾；肩关节放松，肘关节屈曲呈140°，肘部距胸前壁为一拳左右；手指自然弯曲，手背沿掌横弓排列形成弧面(图85，86，87)，以手掌小鱼际缘接触患者体表。

Before drilling the rolling, you ought to hold the right posture as followed. The manipulator stands with two feet separated in front and behind and the upper trunk inclined anteriorly. Relaxes his shoulders, flexes his elbow joint to about 140°, keeps his elbow a fist away from the anterior wall of the thorax, flexes his fingers naturally, and makes the hand back cambered shape along the transverse metacarpal arch (Fig. 85, 86, 87). Then puts the ulnar side of the palm on the patient's body.

在姿势正确的基础上，练习㨰法动作。先将肘关节略伸，前臂前摆旋后，腕关节逐渐掌屈前移，带动手背弧面向前方㨰动，直至第二、三掌骨间隙接触患者体表(图88，89)，紧接着，前臂后摆旋前，腕关节逐渐背伸后移，使手背弧面向后方滚动，直至以手尺侧缘接触体表(图90，91)。将上述操作连续起来，不使间断、停顿，就形成了轻重交替，持续不断的压力波动刺激(图92)。为了便于读者理解㨰法动作形式，图93以机械模型说明之。

When the posture is corrected, one may drill the rolling manipulation. At first, the elbow joint is slightly extended, the forearm is swung anteriorly and supinated, and the wrist joint is relaxed and moved forward gradually. Thus the arch surface of hand back is driven to roll ahead until the interval between the second and the third metacarpal bone touches the body surface(Fig. 88, 89). Immediately, the elbow is flexed slightly, the forearm is swung posterior and pronated, the wrist is extended and moved backward and the hand back is rolled to back until the hypothenar side of the hand touches the body surface(Fig. 90,91). When the above actions are linked without breaking, the manipulation becomes a lasted stimulation that the force is light alternated in strength (Fig. 92). Aiming to making it easy to understand the manipulative manner of the rolling, the Fig. 93 illustrates with a mechanical model.

滚法操作中，使操作者手背弧面在患者体表上形成滚动运动，若二者之间产生相对滑移(拖动)或手背相对体表而空转，都是不对的(图94)。滚法操作过程中，要控制好腕关节的屈伸运动，不使腕关节出现折刀样的突变动作而造成跳动感。滚法操作时也不可有意识地向下用力顶压，压力、频率、摆动幅度要均匀一致，动作协调而有节律性。

During rolling, the back of the manipulator's hand is rolled on the patient's body. Either the manner in which the two touch aspects slide relatively or the back of hand turns without moving forward and backward are not right(Fig. 94). During rolling manipulation, one must control the flexion-extensional movement of the wrist to keep the patient from feeling jumping sensation caused by sudden movement of the wrist as a folding knife. It is also not allowed to press down consciously. The pressing force, frequency and the swinging range ought to be uniform. The action must be harmonious and rhythmical.

滚法的压力大，接触面积也大，刺激刚柔相济，适用于颈项、肩背、腰臀、四肢大关节等肌肉丰厚部位的操作。具有舒筋通络、滑利关节、增强肌肉、韧带活动能力，促进血液循环及消除疲劳的作用。治疗软组织损伤、运动系统与神经系统疾病具有独特的疗效。

The rolling has strong pressing force and large touching area. Its stimulation is both forceful and mild. It is

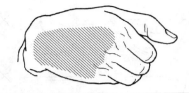

图89　滚法前滚时的接触面
Fig. 89　Touch surface of anterior roll

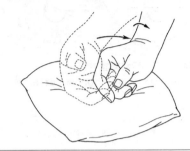

图90　滚法回滚运动
Fig. 90　Posterior roll of rolling

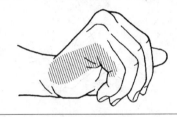

图91　滚法回滚时的接触面
Fig. 91　Touch surface of posterior roll

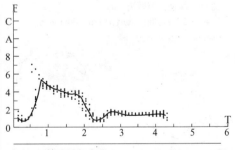

图92　滚法叠加曲线
Fig. 92　Pile-up curve of rolling

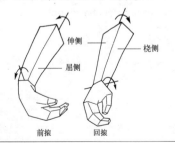

图93　滚法操作机械模型
Fig. 93　Mechanical model of rolling

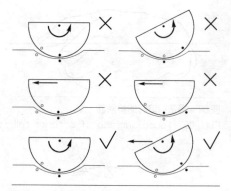

图94 不同的运动类型
Fig. 94 Model of motional patterns

suitable for manipulating on neck, shoulder, back, waist, buttocks and the major joints of limbs where the muscles are well developed. Rolling can relax the muscles and tendons, dredge blocked channels, lubricate joints, enhance the motive ability of the muscle and the ligaments, promote the blood circulation and remove weary. It has unique curative effects on healing the injury of soft tissues, the diseases of the kinetic system and the nervous system.

四、滚法的衍化
Evolution of Rolling

1. 掌指关节滚法

滚法以手背弧面与患者接触，刺激较为柔和舒适。在滚法的推广应用过程中，一些操作者认为以掌指关节骨突形成接触，用腕关节单纯伸屈运动代替腕关节屈伸与前臂旋转的复合运动，能获得更大压力和刺激强度。掌指关节滚法适用于腰背肌僵硬、感觉迟钝者治疗。图95为掌指关节滚法，图96为掌指关节滚法接触面。

1. Rolling with the metacarpo-phalangeal joints

During rolling, the manipulator touches the body surface with the cambered surface of the back of hand, so its stimulation is relatively mild and comfortable to the patient. As the spreading and applying course of the rolling, it was thought that if the bone bulges of the metacarpophalangeal joints are taken to touch body surface and with the simple flexion-extension movement of the wrist instead of the compound movements of the flexion-extension of the wrist and the rotation of forearm, stronger force and stimulation could be achieved. The rolling with the metacarpophalangeal joints is adapted to cure those who suffer from stiff muscles and insensibility on back. The Fig.95 is rolling with the metacarpophalangeal joints, the Fig.96 is its touch surface.

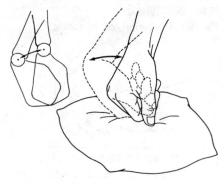

图95 掌指关节滚法
Fig. 95 Rolling with the metacarpo-phalangeal joints

 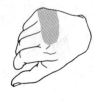

图96 掌指关节滚法接触面
Fig. 96 Touch surface of rolling with the metacarpophalangeal joints

2. 滚法

滚法以示、中、环指近侧指间关节骨突形成接触，通过腕关节屈伸运动使指间关节前后滚动。滚法适用于头部操作，治疗头痛、失眠等症。图97为滚法，图98为滚法接触面。

2. Rolling with the proximal interphalangeal joints

In this rolling, the proximal interphalangeal joints of the index, middle and ring fingers are used to touch body surface and through the flexion–extension of the wrist joint to make the joints rolled forward and backward. Rolling with the proximal interphalangeal joints is adapted to manipulate on head for curing headache, insomnia etc. The Fig. 97 shows the rolling with the proximal interphalangeal joints and the Fig. 98 is its touch surface.

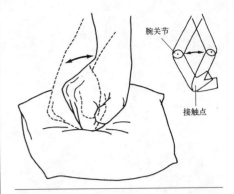

Fig. 97 Rolling with the proximal interphalangeal joints

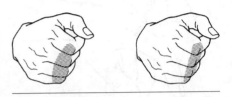

Fig. 98 Touch surface of rolling with the proximal interphalangeal joints

[附] 一指禅推法与滚法练习
[Appendix] The Drilling of Dhyana-Thumb-Pushing and Rolling

1. 一指禅推法练习

一指禅推法操作中，前臂的旋后旋前摆动是其运动形式的主要方面，而拇指的运动则是由前臂摆动、腕部空间位置变化而引起的伴随运动。初学者往往过分重视拇指运动，甚至有意识地屈伸拇指，不但引起大鱼际酸痛，而且把手法练僵。因此，在学习一指禅推法过程中，建议分两步走。第一阶段，操作者主要练习正确的前臂摆动运动，不考虑拇指伴随摆动。可令操作者拇指与示指相贴，虎口闭拢，练习前臂摆动(图99)。第二阶段，在前臂摆动协调、熟练的基础上，再将虎口放松，使拇指与示指在前臂摆动过程中自然出现开合动作。

1. Drill of Dhyana-Thumb-pushing

During the manipulative procedure of the Dhyana-thumb-pushing, the pronation and supination are the main aspects of its action manner. While the motion of the thumb is the accompanied motion caused by the wrist location variation in space due to swinging of the forearm. The learners usually pay over attention to the motion of the thumb, even more, flex and extend the thumb consciously. Thus not only the big thenar eminence is felt pain and sore, but also the manipulation is become inflexible. Because of these, the writer suggest learner to take two steps in the drill process of the dhyana-thumb-pushing. The first step, the learner mainly drills correct swinging motion of the forearm and doesn't consider the passively motion of the thumb. One may close the first web of the hand, keep the thumb against the index

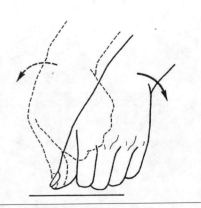

Fig. 99 First step of drill of Dhyana-thumb-pushing

finger, and then swing the forearm to and fro simply (Fig.99). The second step is that, on the basis of harmonious and skilled swinging of the forearm, the manipulator relaxes the first web to make the thumb and the index finger opened and closed during the swinging process of the forearm.

2. 滚法练习

滚法操作中,腕关节的屈伸运动是其运动形式的主要方面。初学者操作错误中,以腕关节屈伸运动不够占大多数,而前臂旋转运动大多存在。因此在学习滚法过程中,作者也建议分两步走。第一步,先练习腕关节屈伸运动,可令操作者一手轻握另一手的手指,使其位置相对固定;先将腕关节前摆,掌屈至极限位,再使腕关节后摆,背伸至40°左右;连续以上操作,勿使中断。此阶段并不形成滚动,而是手小鱼际缘的摩擦滑动(图100)。第二步,在腕关节屈伸摆动熟练、协调的基础上,解除对手指的固定,注意使手背接触部位随前后摆动不断改变,将摩擦运动改为滚动,就自然形成了腕屈伸与前臂旋转的复合运动。

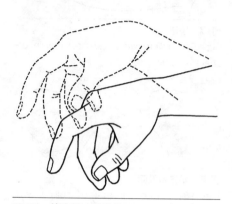

图100 滚法第一阶段练习
Fig. 100 First step of drill of rolling

2. Drill of rolling

The flexion-extension of the wrist is the main aspect of the motion pattern in the rolling manipulation. Among the manipulative errors of the learners, deficiency of flexion-extension of the wrist is accounted for the most, but the rotation of the forearm nearly all exists. So the writer also suggests the learner to take two steps in learning rolling. The first step is to drill the flexion-extension of the wrist as followed. The manipulator holds the fingers of the operating hand with his other hand to fix it in certain location, then swings the wrist forward and flexes it to the limit situation, and then makes the wrist swing backward and extend to about 40°. With linking the above actions without breaking, the drill process becomes smoother and smoother, faster and faster. In fact, during first step, the manipulative manner isn't the rolling movement but rubbing and slipping under the hypothenar side of the hand (Fig.100). On the second step, after achieving harmonious and skilled flexion-extension swing of the wrist, the manipulator removes the fixation of the fingers and makes the touch part of the back of hand be changed constantly. Thus the rubbing movement is replaced with rolling, and the profound movements of the flexion-extension of the wrist and the rotation of the forearm is naturally formed.

第五节　捏拿类手法
SECTION 5 CATEGORY OF PINCHING-GRASPING MANIPULATIONS

所谓捏拿类手法是指以操作者的指、掌从皮肤对称的位置向深部挤压的一类操作。捏拿类手法可以用图101模拟表示。

Category of pinching-grasping refers to those actions in which the manipulator squeezes body tissues from two opposed side with his fingers or palms. These manipulations can be modeled with Fig.101.

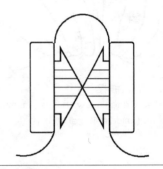

图101　捏拿类手法模式图
Fig. 101 Model of category of pinching-grasping manipulations

一、代表手法　捏法
Principal Techniques of Pinching-Grasping Manipulations: Pinching

以拇指与其他手指相对,将患者皮肤及少量皮下组织捏起,称捏法。捏法常用于小儿脊柱两侧操作,有两种操作方式。

The manipulation in which the manipulator holds the patient's skin and some subcutaneous tissues and pulls them up with the thumb and other fingers oppositely is called as pinching. The pinching is often applied on two sides of infant's spine. There are two different manipulative manners.

1. 拇示指捏
患儿俯卧,使背部肌肉松弛。操作者将两手示指屈曲,以示指中节背面紧触脊柱两侧皮肤,拇指前按皮肤后向后捏起,随捏随提,两手交替向前推进,自龟尾至大椎处(图102,103)。

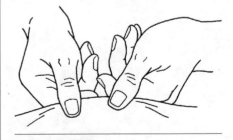

图102　拇示指捏
Fig. 102 Pinching with the thumb and the index finger

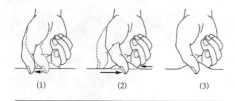

图103 拇示指捏操作分解步骤
Fig. 103 Decomposed steps of pinching with the thumb and index finger

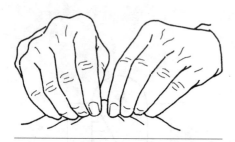

图104 拇示中指捏
Fig. 104 Pinching with the thumb, the index and middle fingers

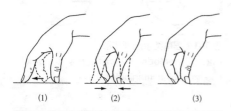

图105 拇示中指捏操作分解步骤
Fig. 105 Decomposed steps of pinching with the thumb, the index and middle fingers

1. Pinching with the thumb and index finger

The suffered infant lies prostrately to make the back muscles to be relaxed. The manipulator touches the paraspinal skin of the infant with the backside of the middle section of the index finger, which is flexed and put behind. Then moves the thumb forward to presses skin and pinches the skin between in the thumb and the index finger. As the skin is pinched, the manipulator pulls it up and then lets it off. This action is done alternately by two hands from the point Guiwei to the point Dazhui (Fig. 102, 103).

2. 拇示中指捏

患儿体位同上。操作者将两手拇指桡侧偏峰紧触脊柱两侧皮肤，示中指前按皮肤后相对捏起。随捏随提，两手交替前进（图104，105）。

2. Pinching with the thumb, the index and middle fingers

The infant's posture is the same as the above. With the thumb putting behind to touch the paraspinal skin, and the index and middle fingers moving forward to press the skin, the manipulator pinches the skin between the thumb and the rest two fingers. Then pulls it up and then lets it off. The two hands move alternately(Fig.104, 105).

捏脊法临床应用范围较广，在小儿推拿中尤为常用。一般认为捏脊法偏于补益，具有调和阴阳，健脾和胃，增强人体抗病能力的作用，治疗小儿疳积、消化不良、腹泻呕吐、体弱多病等病症，也可治疗成人消化道疾患、月经不调、痛经、失眠等症。

The clinical applying range of pinching spine is very broad, it is more frequently used in pediatric Tuina. It is generally believed that the functions of pinching spine incline to nourishing and invigorating. It can balance Yin and Yang, reinforce the spleen and normalize the stomach and strengthen the body resistance. It is used for curing malnutrition and food stagnation in children, indigestion, diarrhea, vomiting and poor health condition. It is also used for curing adult's diseases, such as digestive tract disorders, irregular menstruation, dysmenorrhoea, insomnia etc.

此外，在骨科手法中，也有捏法(图106)，是指操作者以两手掌相对挤压，使骨折碎片向纵轴线靠拢，适用于粉碎性和长斜形骨折、长螺旋形骨折的整复对位。为同名异法，应予分清。

Besides, there is pinching in orthopedic manipulations as well (Fig.106). It is referred to that the manipulator squeezes the limb with his palms oppositely to make the pieces of broken bone close up to the longitudinal axis. It is suitable for correcting fracture such as comminuted fracture, long oblique fracture and long spiral fracture. The two pinching are different in manipulation but same in name, therefore they should be distinguished.

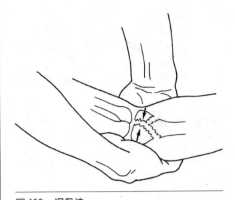

图106　捏骨法
Fig. 106　Pinching of bone setting

二、捏法的衍化
Evolution of Pinching

1. 拿法

拿法与捏法操作非常相似，在命名上也随作者的习惯称呼之，概念不十分清楚。一般而言，捏法是指捏拿皮肤及少量皮下组织的操作。在捏法的基础上，增加捏拿组织的体积和力量，将肌肉连同皮肤、皮下组织一起捏起上提，再让肌肤逐渐从手指间滑出，为拿法(图107，108)。

1. Grasping

The grasping is very similar to the pinching in manipulative manner, Their names are also promiscuous together due to the writers habits in various books. Because the concepts of them are not very clear, in general, the pinching refers to the manipulation in which only the skin and a little subcutaneous tissue are held. While the grasping refers to the manipulation that not only the skin and the subcutaneous tissue are held, but the muscles as well, then the tissues are slipped out of the fingers(Fig.107,108).

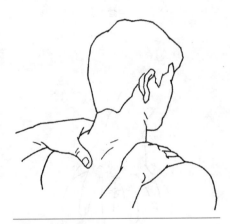

图107　拿法
Fig. 107　Grasping

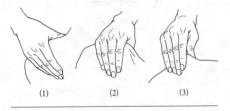

图108　拿法操作分解步骤
Fig. 108　Decomposed steps of grasping

拿法刺激性较强，故提拿时，手指应伸直，以平坦的指面着力于肌肉，类似夹子的动作(图109)。不可将手指屈曲，以尖锐的指端着力，形成钳子样的动作，以免患者感觉不舒适。

The stimulation of grasping is relatively stronger. So

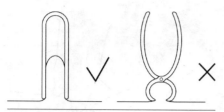

图109 拿法操作模式
Fig. 109 Manipulative model of grasping

you ought to straighten the fingers and put the flat finger-print regions on the skin. This action is like the action of a clip(Fig.109). You mustn't flex your fingers and put the sharp fingernails on the skin to come into pincerlike action. Thus the patient can avoid uncomfortable sensation.

拿法操作时，腕部放松，捏拿动作连绵不断，用力由轻到重，由重到轻。拿法适用于颈项、肩部和四肢肌肉丰厚处操作，具有疏通经络、放松肌肉、解表发汗、止痛活血的作用，治疗头痛项强、关节痹痛、肌肉酸胀、感冒等症。

During the grasping manipulation, the wrist is relaxed, the pinching-grasping action is uninterrupted, the power is changed from mild to strong and from strong to weak. Grasping is adapted on the neck, shoulder and limb regions where the muscles are developed. It has the abilities to dredge blocked channel and collateral, relax the muscle, relieve superficial syndrome by means of diaphoresis, relieve pain and invigorate the blood circulation. Those illnesses such as headache, stiff neck, arthrilgia, muscle sore, cold etc. can be treated by grasping.

2. 抓法

捏法、拿法是将拇指与其他手指从轴对称位置自两侧向中线挤法。若将五指从辐射对称位置自四周向中心挤压，则为抓法(图110)。抓法在临床上较为少用，仅作为辅助手法。适用于头部、腹部操作，治疗头痛、腹痛等症。

2. Seizing

Both in pinching and grasping, the manipulator compresses the tissues from both sides to the middle line with thumb and other fingers. If one compressed from several points to the central point with fingers, this manipulation is called as seizing(Fig.110). Seizing is a supplementary manipulation and is not so frequently used as pinching and grasping in clinic. It is suitable for manipulation on head, abdominal regions to cure headache and abdominal pain.

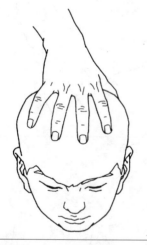

图110 抓法
Fig. 110 Seizing

3. 弹筋法

拿法用力提捏肌肤后，逐渐松开手指，让肌肤慢慢滑回原处。若用力提捏肌肤后，立即松开手指，使紧张的肌肤迅速弹回原处，则称为弹筋法(图 111)。弹筋法有剥离粘连、解除肌肉痉挛的作用，适用于肌腹、肌腱部位操作。

3. Plucking tendon

During grasping manipulation, the fingers are gradually loosened to let the skin and muscles off the original situation, after the skin and muscles are held and pulled. If the fingers are loosened immediately to make the strained skin and muscles be jumped to original situation swiftly as the skin and muscles are held and pulled, the manipulation is called as plucking tendon (Fig.111). The plucking tendon is able to peel off adherence and relieve muscle convulsion and is suitable for manipulation on muscles and tendons.

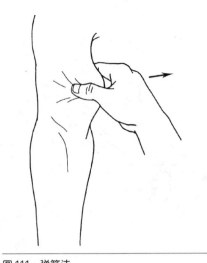

图 111　弹筋法
Fig. 111　Plucking tendon

4. 挤法

捏法挤压皮肤、皮下组织的力量很轻，一般以不引起痛苦为限，且捏挤的部位不断移动。若拇、示二指相对挤捏的力量很重，且重复在同一部位操作，直至皮下血管破裂，出现瘀血，则称为挤法，又称为挤痧(图 112)。

4. Squeezing

The force of pinching is very mild. Generally, the limitation is controlled not to cause pain, and the pinching points are always moved. If the compressing force of the thumb and index finger is stronger, and the action is repeated at the same site until the subcutaneous vessels are broken and some petechiae appeared, the manipulation is named for squeezing, or named for squeezing "Sha"(Fig.112).

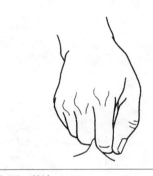

图 112　挤法
Fig. 112　Squeezing

5. 扯法

在挤法的基础上，再增加上提皮肤的操作，直至皮下瘀血，则称扯法，或称扯痧(图 113)。

5. Tearing

On the basis of the squeezing manipulation, if one repeats to do the action of pulling until some petechiae appears under the subcutaneous tissues, the manipulation is named for tearing or tearing "Sha"(Fig.113).

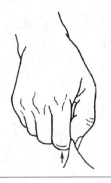

图 113　扯法
Fig. 113　Tearing

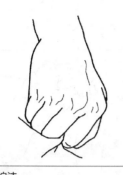

图114 拧法
Fig. 114 Twisting (Turning)

6. 拧法

又称扭法。以弯曲的示、中指近侧指间关节处捏起皮肤后，左右扭转，使皮下瘀血，亦称拧痧、扭痧(图114)。挤、扯、拧、扭法都是民间治疗痧证的一些手法，常在额面部、鼻梁、颈项部、胸部、脊椎两侧、肘窝、腘窝处操作，具有开通气机，发散病邪，开窍醒神的作用，对许多内科急症有很好的疗效。

6. Twisting

It was also named as turning. In twisting, the manipulator pinches the skin with flexed proximal interphalangeal joints of the index and middle fingers, then twists the skin rightward and leftward to make some petechiae be appeared within the subcutaneous tissue. It is also named for twisting "Sha" or turning "Sha"(Fig. 114). Squeezing, tearing, twisting, and turning are all the folk methods to be used for infections in early stage. They are often adapted on the forehead, bridge of the nose, neck and nape, chest, paraspinal region, hollow of the elbow, hollow of the knee. They have the effects of ventilating Qi, dispersing ill evil and regaining consciousness. And a lot of internal emergencies showed good responses to them.

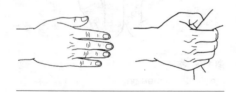

图115 挪法
Fig. 115 Shifting

7. 挪法

手掌平置于腹部，然后如握拳状将腹壁抓紧提起片刻，再松开手掌稍向前移，再抓提腹壁，不断地前移，直至整个腹部操作一遍(图115)。本法刺激强烈，用于小儿蛔虫性肠梗阻、肠粘连等症的治疗。

7. Shifting

Putting the hand on the abdomen, the manipulator holds the abdomen as holding fists and pulls it up, then loosens the hand and moves forward a bit and repeats the above actions until the whole abdomen has been acted thoroughly(Fig. 115). This manipulation stimulation is strong and is applied to treat intestinal obstruction due to ascariasis of the children and the intestinal adhesion.

8. 合法

两手掌对置关节对称位置，同时向关节纵轴相对挤压合拢，称合法或归合法。合法为理筋手法，常用于关节软组织损伤，如下尺桡关节分离的治疗(图 116)。

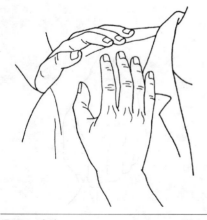

图116 合法
Fig. 116 Concentrating

8. Concentrating

Two hands are put on the opposite locations of a joint to squeeze it so as to concentrate the separated joint. This manipulation is called as concentrating or concentrating reduction. This manipulation belongs to the manipulations of arranging tendon. It is usually applied to cure the soft tissue injury of joint. For example, the distal radioulnar joint separation(Fig.116).

三、复合手法
Compound-manipulations

1. 捏揉法、拿揉法
在揉法、拿法基础上，配合手指的揉捻动作，则称为捏揉法或拿揉法(图117)。

1. Pinching-kneading, Grasping-kneading
On the basis of pinching or grasping manipulation and coordinating with kneading and twisting action, the manipulation becomes pinching-kneading or grasping-kneading (Fig.117).

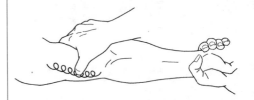

图117　捏揉法
Fig. 117　Pinching-kneading

2. 捻法
在捏手指、足趾时，配合揉捻动作和指间关节、掌指关节的扭转运动，称捻法(图118)。捻法用于治疗指、趾疼痛，指间关节扭伤。

2. Holding-kneading
If one kneads and rotates a finger or toe with two or three fingers, the manipulation is called as holding-kneading(Fig.118). The holding-kneading is applied to cure finger or toe pain and the interphalangeal joint sprain.

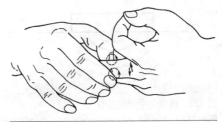

图118　捻法
Fig. 118　Holding-kneading

3. 搓法
在合法的基础上，配合手掌环转揉动，并沿肢体纵轴上下移动，为搓法(图119)。搓法常用于四肢、腰部、胁肋部操作，作为结束手法使用，有放松肌肉、减轻疼痛、促进血液循环的作用。

3. Rubbing with two palms
Rubbing with two palms refers to concentrating ma-

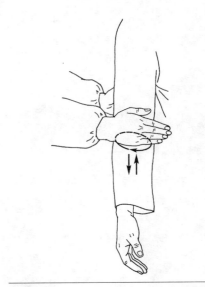

图119　搓法
Fig. 119　Rubbing with two palms

nipulation coordinated with circular rubbing and shifting the palms along axis of the limb (Fig. 119). It is often used on the limbs, back and rib regions and as a final manipulation. It can relax muscles, relieve pain and promote the blood circulation.

第六节 振动类手法
SECTION 6 CATEGORY OF VIBRATING MANIPULATIONS

所谓振动类手法是指以指、掌轻触患者体表后，通过肌肉快速、小幅度运动产生较高频率的震颤，并将震颤波动传递给患者肌肤的一类操作(图120)。

The so-called "Category of vibration manipulation" means those actions in which the fingers or palms are put on the patient's body slightly, then some higher frequency vibration produced by speedy and fine muscle motion of the manipulator is transmitted to the patient's tissues(Fig.120).

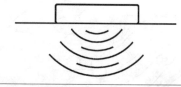

图 120 振动类手法模式图
Fig. 120 Model of category of vibrating manipulation

一、代表手法 振法
Principal Techniques of Vibrating Manipulations: Vibrating

振法根据操作者接触部位的不同而分为掌振法和指振法两种，但其姿势、操作方式基本相似。操作者肩关节外展30°左右，肘关节屈曲约140°。

The vibrating manipulations are divided into two manipulative manners, vibrating with palm and vibrating with fingers, according to the touch parts. But, their postures, manipulative manners are very similar. The manipulator abducts his shoulder about 30° and flexes his elbow about 140°

1. 指振法

垂腕，手指自然伸直，以示、中两指指端轻触患者一定穴位(图121)。

1. Vibrating with the fingers

The manipulator flexes the wrist, extends the fingers naturally and puts the tip of the index and middle finger at a point of the patient's body gently (Fig.121).

2. 掌振法

腕关节略背伸，手指自然伸直，以手掌面轻按于患者体表某部位(图122)。

2. Vibrating with the palm

The manipulator extends the wrist slightly, the fingers naturally and puts the palm on a part of the patient's body gently (Fig.122).

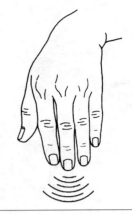

图121. 指振法
Fig. 121 Vibrating with the fingers

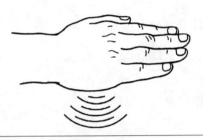

图122. 掌振法
Fig. 122 Vibrating with the palm

然后，操作者可用两种不同的运动方式产生高频振动。一种为痉挛性肌震颤方式，前臂和手部肌肉强烈地作静止性收缩，产生振颤动作，振动频率可达每分钟600~800次。本法容易学习，但由于肌肉持续痉挛，影响本身血液循环，很快疲劳。第二种为交替性肌收缩振动，操作者肌肉放松，前臂屈肌和伸肌作快速交替性收缩，但不产生明显的手部运动，而是产生细微振动，振动频率一般为每分钟300~400次。本法掌握困难，但由于肌肉交替地收缩、舒张，血液循环不受影响，不易疲劳。

Then the higher frequency vibration may be created with two different manners of muscle motion. A sort of them is the convulsive manner. During this manner, the muscles of the arm are kept in static contraction intensely to bring about thrill. The vibration frequency can reach as high as 600 to 800 times per minute. This manner is easily to be learned, but quickly tired because of the muscles contraction that may block the blood circulation of the muscles. The other is alternated contraction manner of muscle. Under this manipulative manner, the flexion and extension muscles make speedy contraction or dilatation in turn to engender fine thrill without obvious hand moving. The vibration frequency is about 300 to 400 times per minute. The later manner is difficult to be held, but more durable, since the muscle contracting and relaxing are alternated and the blood circulation is not obviously affected.

振法操作的能量消耗较大,应保持自然呼吸,切忌憋气,以免影响操作者自身健康。也可在操作时将意念集中于操作部位上,即所谓"运气推拿"。本法可使局部产生温热舒适感,多用于脘腹胀痛、消化不良、中气下陷等症的辅助治疗,具有健脾消积,调节胃肠蠕动的功能。

Since the energy consumption of the vibrating manipulation is higher, one should keep in natural breath and avoid holding respiration, so as to free from impair in one's health. That the manipulator keeps his idea on the acted part of the patient is also allowed in vibrating manipulation. Thus is so called "Tuina of Transferring Qi". Vibrating manipulation can cause the local tissues to feel warm and comfortable. It is usually applied to the supplementary manipulation for fullness and pain in epigastric and abdominal regions, indigestion and descended Qi in middle Jiao. It has such functions as invigorating the spleen, removing stagnant food, regulating the gastrointestinal peristalsis etc.

二、振法的衍化 摆法
Evolution of the Vibrating: Waving

振法所产生的振动是上下波动,若改变振动的方向,使波动向周围传导,则成为摆法。摆法操作时,以手尺侧缘置患者体表,腕关节放松,然后作快速小幅度的摆腕动作(腕屈伸动作),带动体表组织产生高频振动(图123)。摆法适用于胸腹、腰背、四肢部位的操作,具有放松肌肉,调和脾胃,促进血液循环,缓急止痛的作用,治疗消化不良、肌肉痉挛、局部肿痛等症。

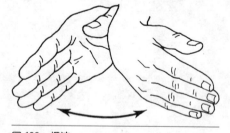

图123 摆法
Fig.123 Waving

The vibration of the vibrating manipulation is oscillated up and down. If the direction of vibration is changed to surrounding area transversely, the manipulation is called as waving. When the waving is done, the ulnar side of the hand is put on the patient's body with his wrist joint relaxed. Then the manipulator makes speedy and minor ringed movement of flexion and extension of wrist to cause the superficial tissues of the patient's body to generate high frequency vibration (Fig.123). The waving is adapted to be manipulated on the chest, abdomen and limb regions. It has the effects of relaxing the muscles, regulating the digestive function, promoting the blood circulation, alleviating spasm and relieving pain. It is often used to cure indigestion, muscle convulsion and swelling pain on local tissue.

三、复合手法
Compound Manipulations

1. 提颤法
本法为捏拿与振动的复合手法。手指分开呈半屈状态，以拇指与示指、中指轻轻捏提肌肤后，腕、指作快速颤抖动作，两手交替操作(图124)。本法具有放松肌肉、活血化瘀止痛、分离粘连的作用，适用于颈项、四肢及腹部操作。

1. Lifting-trembling
This manipulation is a compound manipulation combined grasping with vibrating. With opening the fingers to form semiflexion condition, the manipulator holds the patient's skin and muscles gently with the thumb, the index and middle fingers. Then makes the wrist and the fingers tremble quickly. This manipulation can be done with the two hands one by one (Fig.124). This manipulation has the functions of relaxing muscles, promoting blood circulation and removing blood stasis, relieving pain, separating adhesion and so on. It is suitable for manipulated on the neck, limb and abdominal regions.

2. 荡法
在提颤法的基础上，增加左右上下颤动的运动幅度，降低颤抖频率，则称为荡法(图125)。本法仅用于腹部操作，具有消积利气，分离粘连的作用，治疗小儿蛔虫团肠梗阻、肠粘连等症。

2. Swinging
Based on the lifting-trembling manipulation, the so

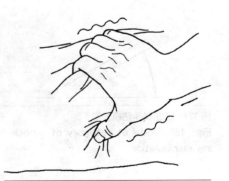

图124 提颤法
Fig. 124 Lifting-trembling

called swinging required the manipulator to increase the movement range of trembling but reducing the frequency (Fig.125). The manipulation is only used on the abdomen. It has the effects to remove stagnant food, smooth Qi, separate adhesion. It is adapted to treat ascarid ileus of children and intestinal adhesion etc.

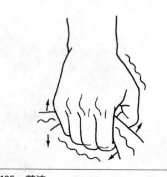

图 125 荡法
Fig. 125 Swinging

3. 对掌振法

本法为合法与振法的复合手法。两手掌分置于关节的对称部位，然后作快速上下(或左右)振颤动作。本法适用于四肢关节的操作(图126)。

3. Concentrating-Vibrating

This manipulation is the compound manipulation combined concentrating with vibrating. Two palms are put on the symmetrical side of the joint and then speedy trembling that is vibrated up and down (or left and right) is produced. This manipulation is suitable for manipulating on the joints of the limbs(Fig. 126).

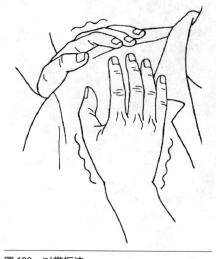

图 126 对掌振法
Fig. 126 Concentrating-vibrating

第七节 叩击类手法

SECTION 7 CATEGORY OF KNOCKING MANIPULATIONS

所谓叩击类手法是指以指、掌、拳或器具对患者体表进行有节律地、间断地击打的一类操作(图127)。

Category of knocking manipulation means those actions during which the manipulator knocks the patient's body rhythmically and disconnectedly with one's finger, palm, fist or tools (Fig.127).

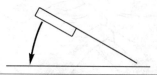

图 127 叩击类手法模式图
Fig. 127 Model of category of knocking manipulation

一、代表手法 击法
Principal Techniques of the Knocking Manipulation: Knocking

以较重的力量单次或多次击打某一体表部位，使击打力量作用到肌肉、骨骼等深部组织，称击法。击法可用拳、掌，也可用特制的棒(桑枝棒)，故击法有以下不同的操作方式。

The manipulation in which the manipulator knocks a point of the patient's body for one time or several times with relatively strong force to make power impact into the muscles, bone etc. deep tissues is called as knocking. Both some parts of human body such as the fist, palm, finger and tools such as a stick made of mulberry twigs can be used in knocking. The knocking has the below different manipulative manners.

1. 拳背击

手握空拳，腕关节伸直，以肘部发力，将拳背有节律地反复击打某一部位；或边击打，边移动作用部位(图128)。拳背击适用于肩背部操作。

1. Knocking with the fist back

Holding an empty fist, extending the wrist joint, the manipulator knocks at the patient's body surface with the fist back by the means of delivering force from the elbow rhythmically and repeatedly. Or changes the acting points while knocking (Fig.128). This manipulation is adapted to the shoulder and back regions.

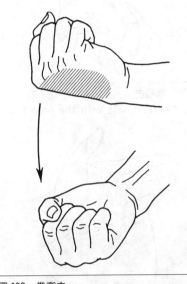

图 128 拳背击
Fig. 128 Knocking with the fist back

2. 捶击

手握空拳，腕关节放松，以肘部发力，将两拳尺侧缘交替捶击某一部位，捶击法用力一般要比拳背击轻。捶击法适用于肩背、四肢部位操作(图129)。

2. Thumping

The thumping requires the manipulator to hold two empty fists, relax the wrists, then knock at a point with the ulnar sides of the fists in turn by the means of delivering force from the elbow. The force of thumping is generally lighter than that of the knocking with the fist back. The thumping is usually applied on the shoulder, back and limb regions (Fig.129).

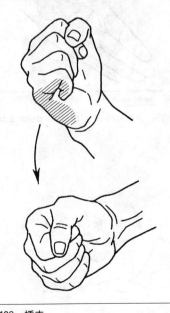

图 129 捶击
Fig. 129 Thumping

3. 掌根击

手指微屈，腕关节背伸至极限位，然后以肩关节发力，将掌根部反复击打某一部位；或边击打，边移动击打部位。掌根击适用于臀部及大腿肌肉丰厚处操作（图130）。

3. Knocking with the palm heel

The manipulator extends the fingers, relaxes the wrist, and knocks at the patient's body surface with the palm heel by the means of delivering force from the shoulder rhythmically and repeatedly. This manipulation is suited to be manipulated on the buttock and the thigh where the muscles are well grew(Fig. 130).

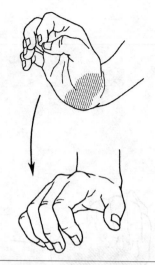

图130 掌根击
Fig. 130 Knocking with the palm heel

4. 掌侧击

手指伸直，腕关节放松，然后以腕关节发力，用手掌尺侧缘反复击打某一部位（图131）。本法形如刀劈，故又称劈法，适用于肩背、四肢关节及指(趾)缝处操作。

4. Knocking with the palm edge

The manipulation requires the manipulator to extend the fingers, relax the wrist and then knocks at the patient's body surface with the palm edge by the means of delivering force from the wrist rhythmically and repeatedly (Fig.131).This manipulative form is like chopping with a knife. Therefore it is also named as chopping.This manipulation is suitable for the shoulder, back, joints of the limbs and the cracks between fingers or toes.

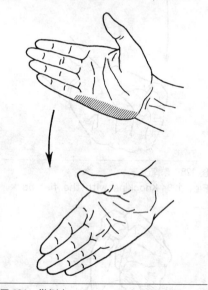

图131 掌侧击
Fig. 131 Knocking with the palm edge

5. 棒击

手握桑枝棒（略有弹性）的一端，腕关节放松，然后视需要，以肘关节发力（力量较轻）或肩关节发力（力量较大），用棒身连续在某一部位击打3～5下（图132），再移动击打部位。棒击时，力量要由轻而重，适可而止；击打的方向应与肌肉、骨骼平行，棒身接触部位应尽可能大，不要用棒尖打，也不要打出头棒（图133）。

5. Knocking with the stick

During this manipulation, the manipulator hold one end of a stick made of mulberry twigs (it is slightly elastic), relax the wrist and then knocks at the patient's body surface with the stick by the means of delivering force from the elbow (it is slighter),or from the shoulder

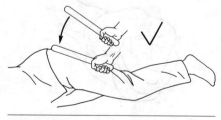

图132 棒击
Fig. 132 Knocking with the stick

(it is stronger), rhythmically and repeatedly for 3 to 5 times, according to clinical condition(Fig.132). Then moves the impacting point while knocking, the force should be changed from light to strong but not too heavy. The stick axis should be parallel to the muscles and bones. The touch part of stick should be as large as possible. It isn't allowed to knock with the stick tip or to make the stick tip out of the patient's body (Fig.133).

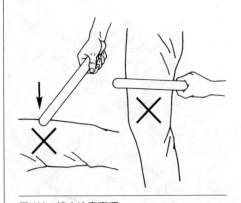

图133 棒击注意事项
Fig. 133 Note items on knocking with the stick

击法力量较大,击打过程中不能有拖拉现象;击打过程要短促,一触即弹起,避免造成组织损伤。击法的操作频率为每分钟45～80次。

The force of the knocking is strong. During the knocking procedure, one mustn't haul the stick while knocking. The knocking procedure should be brief, and spring up immediately after the stick knocking on the body so as to avoid injury of the tissue. The manipulation frequency is 45 to 80 times per minute.

击法适用于肌肉丰厚处操作。具有开窍醒神,活血和营通络的作用。治疗头目眩晕,肢体顽麻等证,也可用于体育比赛前运动员精神状态的调整。

The knocking is suitable for manipulation on those parts where are rich with muscles. It plays the roles of refreshing the mind, restoring consciousness, promoting blood circulation and dredging channels. It is often used to treat dizziness and persistent apathetic of limbs. It is also used to regularize the sportsman's spiritual condition before competition.

二、击法的衍化
Evolution of Knocking

1. 叩法
在击法的基础上减轻击打力量,使其作用传达于皮下组织、肌肉;并加快击打频率,使之达到每分钟80～100次,则称为叩法。有以下的操作变化。

1. Tapping
Based on the knocking manipulation, if the force is

reduce to take its effect arrive only at the subcutaneous tissues and the muscles, and the frequency increased up to 80 to 100 times per minute, the manipulation is called as tapping. There are following varies.

(1)合掌叩: 两手手指伸直、并拢、相合，然后以掌尺侧缘快速击打某一部位(图134)。合掌叩适用于肩背、胸胁部位操作。

(1)Tapping with closed palms: With his fingers being extended, adducted and closed, the manipulator taps a part of the body with the ulnar sides of the palms (Fig. 134). This manipulation is suitable on the shoulder, back and thoracic regions.

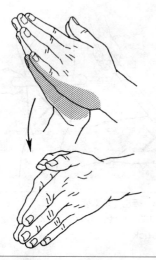

图134. 合掌叩
Fig. 134 Tapping with closed palms

(2)屈指叩: 手指半屈曲，以示、中指近侧指间关节背面轻快地叩击某一部位(图135)。屈指叩适合于小儿推拿操作。

(2)Tapping with flexed fingers: With his fingers being semi-flexed, the manipulator taps a part of the body with the backs of the proximal interphalangeal joints of the index and middle fingers briskly(Fig.135). This tapping is suitable for pediatric Tuina.

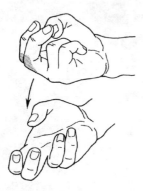

135. 屈指叩
Fig. 135 Tapping with flexed fingers

叩法操作轻快，具有舒松筋脉，促进血液循环，消除疲劳，镇静安神的作用，用于精神紧张、失眠的治疗及体育比赛后的恢复。

The tapping is brisk in manipulating. It possesses the effects of relaxing muscles and tendons, promoting blood circulation, relieving tiredness, tranquilizing the mind and allaying excitement, and is applied to treat stress and insomnia, as well as restore energy after sport competition.

2. 拍法

掌根击与掌侧击都是以手掌着实地击打，若以虚掌轻快地击打，则称拍法。其法：五指并拢，掌心凹陷成虚掌，腕关节放松；然后以腕关节力量，轻快地击打体表(图136)。拍法常用于肩背、腰骶及四肢关节处操作，且有舒松筋脉，促进血液循环的作用。

2. Patting

The manipulator is required to knock the body solidly both in knocking with palm heel and palm edge

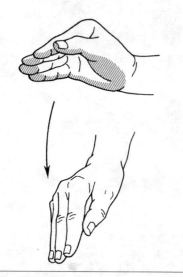

图136 拍法
Fig. 136 Patting

manipulations. If one strikes the body with a hollow palm briskly, the manipulation is called as patting. The manipulator closes the fingers to make a hollow palm, then knocks at the patient's body surface briskly by the means of wrist movement(Fig.136). The patting is usually applied on the shoulder, back, sacrum and limb regions. It can relax the muscles and tendons, promote the blood circulation.

3. 啄法

以五指指尖轻快地击打一定部分，两手交替操作，犹如鸡啄米状，故称啄法。啄法操作既可手指分开如爪状（图137），也可互相聚拢成梅花状（图138）。啄法适用于头面部操作，有安神醒脑的作用，用于头痛、失眠的治疗。

3. Pecking

The manipulator takes the fingers tips of two hands to knock the body briskly and alternatively. Because this manipulation is like the pecking movement of a chicken, it is called as pecking. Either manipulative manners in which the fingers tips are opened as a bird talon (Fig. 137) or closed as a plum is allowed (Fig. 138). The pecking is suited for manipulating on the head and face. It possesses the effects of tranquilizing the mind, restoring consciousness and is applied to treat the headache and insomnia.

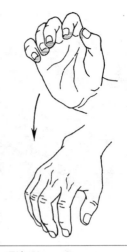

图 137　啄法(1)
Fig. 137　Pecking(1)

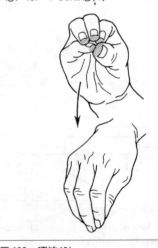

图 138　啄法(2)
Fig. 138　Pecking (2)

4. 弹法

啄法以腕关节力量击打，弹法则是用伸指肌的弹力进行击打。弹法操作即可用示指指腹抵住中指指甲（图139），也可用拇指指腹抵住中指指甲（图140），然后中指迅速弹出，以指尖击打某一穴位。弹法适用于头面部操作，作用同啄法。

4. Flicking

The power of the wrist is used in pecking manipulation, while the elastic force of the extensor of the fingers is delivered in flicking manipulation. That the print region of the index finger contracts on the middle finger nail (Fig.139) and that the thumb print contracts on the middle fingernail are both allowed (Fig.140). Then the middle finger pops swiftly to knock a point with the fingertip. The flicking is suited for manipulation on the

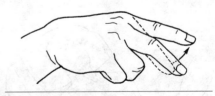

图 139　弹法(1)
Fig. 139　Flicking(1)

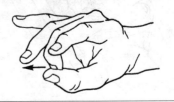

图 140　弹法(2)
Fig. 140　Flicking(2)

head and face. Its function is like the pecking.

拍法、啄法、弹法的操作频率为每分钟100~120次。

The frequency of the patting, pecking and flicking are 100 to 120 times per minute.

第八节 托插类手法
SECTION 8 CATEGORY OF SUPPORTING-INSERTING MANIPULATIONS

所谓托插类手法是指以掌指着力于某部位后向水平方向用力的一类操作(图141)。

The so-called "category of the supporting-inserting manipulation" means those actions in which the manipulator contacts a part of the body with hand, then delivers force in the parallel direction to the body surface(Fig. 141).

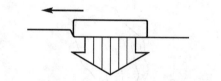

图141 托插类手法模式图
Fig. 141 Model of category of supporting-inserting manipulation

一、代表手法 托法
Principal Techniques of Supporting-inserting Manipulations: Supporting

患者仰卧。操作者将示、中、环、小指伸直并拢，在腹部触及下垂之胃大弯轮廓后，以手指罗纹面与掌小鱼际缘着力，托住胃大弯，顺着患者深吸气运动，将胃大弯沿逆时针方向上托(图142)。本法用于胃下垂的治疗，有益气健脾，提升胃腑的作用。

The patient is in the supine position. The physician extends and closes his four fingers. After having found out the outline of the greater curvature of stomach by palpation on the abdomen, he holds the greater curva-

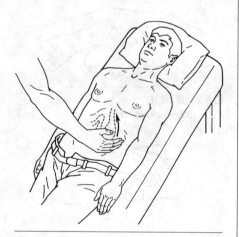

图142 托法
Fig. 142 Supporting

ture of stomach with the print regions of the fingers and the ulnar rim of the palm to support it up in the anticlockwise direction during the patient's deep inhalation period(Fig.142).This manipulation is applied to treat the gastroptosis.Its functions are profiting Qi, invigorating the spleen and raising the stomach level.

二、其他手法
Other manipulations

1. 插法

患者坐位,操作者以左手扶持患者左肩部,右手示、中、环、小指伸直并拢。嘱病人深呼吸,将手指从左侧肩胛骨内下缘向外上方插进,吸气时插入,呼气时稍退出,进退3~5次(图143)。本法也有提升胃腑的作用,用于胃下垂的治疗。

1. Inserting

The patient is in sitting position.The physician holds the left shoulder of the patient with his left hand, extends and closes his four fingers of right hand, then inserts his fingers into the interval between the scapula and chest wall from its medial rim directed lateriorly and superiorly. Then asks the patient to take deep breath. During the inhalation period, his finger tips are inserted deeper and the exhalation period retreated a little.The manipulation can be endured 3 to 5 respiratory periods (Fig.143).This manipulation also has the effect of raising stomach level and is used to treat the gastroptosis.

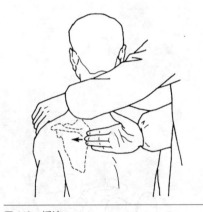

图143 插法
Fig. 143 Inserting

2. 勾法

患者仰卧。操作者两手示、中、环指略屈曲,以指尖勾住肋弓下缘;然后嘱患者深呼吸,操作者手指随呼吸运动而变化勾顶力量,吸气时加重,呼气时减轻(图144)。勾法具有疏肝理气,和胃利胆的作用,治疗胁肋疼痛,脘腹胀痛,消化不良等症。

2. Hooking

The patient is in the supine position. The manipulator flexes the index, middle and ring fingers and hook the inferior rim of the patient's coastal arc with finger tips. Then asks the patient to take deep breath. The hooking

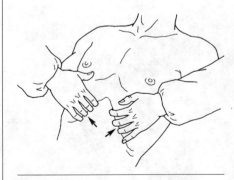

图144 勾法
Fig. 144 Hooking

stimulation is changed stronger during the inhalation period and slighter during the exhalation period (Fig. 144). The hooking is able to smooth the liver Qi, regulate the circulation of Qi, comfort the stomach and profit the gallbladder. It is applied to treat those syndromes such as pain in the hypochondrium, fullness pain in the epigastric regions and indigestion etc.

第九节　环摇类手法
SECTION 9 CATEGORY OF ROTATING MANIPULATIONS

所谓环摇类手法是指由操作者对病变关节作缓和回旋的环旋摇动的一类操作(图145)，属松动性手法范畴。

The so-called "category of the rotating manipulation" means those actions in which the manipulator inducts the patient's suffered joints to be rotated slowly and mildly. It belongs to mobilizing manipulation.

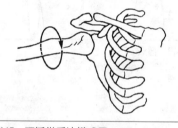

图145　环摇类手法模式图
Fig. 145　Model of Category of Rotating Manipulation

环摇类手法操作时，通常以一手稳定被摇关节近端的肢体，另一手握住被摇关节的远端肢体，根据被摇关节的生理、病理活动范围，以稳妥缓和的力，带动关节作环转运动。关节运动的幅度，应由小到大，逐渐增强，可超过关节病理限制位，但一般不超过其生理限制范围。严禁粗暴动作和违反正常生理活动的运动。

When the category of the rotating manipulations is being done, the manipulator usually takes one hand to stabilize the proximal part of the joint and the other hand to hold the distal part. Then inducts the joint to be rotated with steady and gentle force. The motion breadths should be restricted within the physiological and pathological motion range. The rotation margin should be varied from narrower to broader and increased gradually. It is allowed to exceed the pathological limit, but it mustn't be allowed to exceed the physiological limit. Both violent actions and those actions that transgress the physiological motion manner are strictly forbidden.

一、摇颈
Rotating of the Neck

1. 坐位摇颈

患者坐位，颈项放松，略前屈。操作者用一手扶住其顶枕部，另一手托住下颏，双手协同将头摇转，顺时针与逆时针方向各5~7次（图146）。注意，环摇时不可将头过度后伸。

1. Rotating of the neck in sitting position

The sufferer is in the sitting position, relaxes and flexes his neck slightly. The physician holds the patient's parieto-occipital region with one of his hands and supports patient's chin with the other hand, then inducts the patient's head and neck at the clockwise and anticlockwise directions with placidly force. The above manipulation is repeated for 5 to 7 times in each direction (Fig.146). One should pay attention that it isn't allowed to overextend the head during rotation.

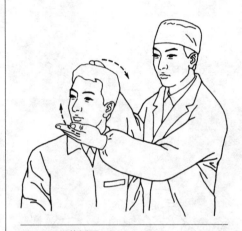

图146 坐位摇颈
Fig. 146 Rotating of the neck in sitting position

2. 卧位摇颈

患者仰卧。操作者站于其头端，先以右前臂伸侧托起患者枕部，右手则抓住患者左肩部，虎口朝向外侧；左手扶住患者头顶；然后利用右前臂的摆动，带动患者头颈作顺时针方向环转摇动3~5周。再交换一下左右手，以左前臂托起患者枕部，右手扶患者头顶，作逆时针方向环摇3~5周（图147）。注意，摇动的动作不能太快，幅度不可过大，以免引起患者眩晕。

2. Rotating of the neck in supine position

The sufferer lies in the supine position. The physician stands at the patient's headend, supports the patient's occiput with his right forearm and grasps patient's left shoulder with the right hand, while holding the patient's headtop with the left hand. Then inducts the patient's head and neck to be rotated at the clockwise direction with placidly force. Then exchanges the role of

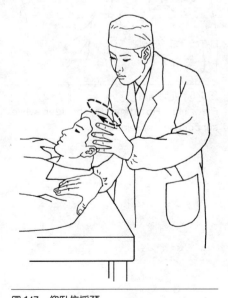

图147 仰卧位摇颈
Fig. 147 Rotating of the neck in supine position

left and right hand to do the same rotating. at the anti-clockwise direction. The above rotation is repeated for 5 to 7times in each direction(Fig.147) One should pay attention to that it isn't allowed to overextend the head during rotation,so as to avoid dizziness.

仰卧位摇颈法操作较稳定，同时限制了颈部后伸运动的幅度，较为安全。适用于颈项疼痛僵硬、活动不利的治疗。

The rotating of neck in supine position is relatively steady, and its restricts the range of extension in the meantime. So it is safer.These manipulations are adapted to heal pain and stiff in neck and inconvenient motion of the neck.

二、摇肩
Rotating of the Shoulder

1. 托肘摇肩

患者坐位，肩部放松。操作者站于其患侧，成弓箭步站立；一手按于肩关节后方，稳定肩部，另一手托起患者屈曲之肘关节，并使患者前臂搁置于自己前臂之上；然后带动患者肩关节作顺时针方向与逆时针方向环转运动各5～10次（图148）。本法操作时，按肩部之手可配合刺激肩部穴位，以减轻环转肩部可能引起的疼痛。本法适用于肩关节疼痛，抬举不利，关节运动障碍较严重者的治疗。

1. Rotating of the shoulder while supporting the elbow

The patient is in the sitting position with relaxed shoulder. With standing on the suffered side in the posture of the forward lunge, the physician puts one hand on the posterior side of the shoulder to stabilize it, supports the flexed elbow and the forearm with his other hand and forearm. Then inducts the shoulder joint to be rotated annularly at the clockwise and anti-clockwise direction for 5 to 10 circles each direction(Fig.148).During this manipulation,the hand that put on the shoulder may cooperate to stimulate the acupoints on the shoulder region, so as to relieve pain caused by rotation motion. The manipulation is suitable for those serious patients who have the troubles of shoulder pain, inconvenient

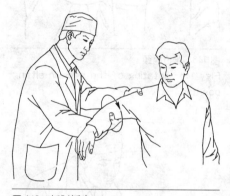

图148 托肘摇肩

Fig. 148 Rotating of shoulder while supporting the elbow

movement of the shoulder.

2. 握手摇肩

患者体位同上。操作者亦以一手扶住其肩关节后上方，另一手握住其手掌，然后带动患者肩关节作顺时针方向与逆时针方向的环转运动各5～10次(图149)。本法操作时，扶肩关节之手可配合刺激肩部穴位，以减轻运动痛。适应范围同上。

2. Rotating of the shoulder while holding the hand

The patient's position is same as the above. The physician puts one hand on the posterior superior part of the shoulder and holds the patient's hand with the other hand. Then inducts the patient's shoulder to be rotated at the both clockwise and anti-clockwise direction for 5 to 10 circles(Fig.149). During this manipulation, the hand that puts on the shoulder may cooperate to stimulate the acupoints so as to relieve pain caused by motion. The scope of application is the same as the above one.

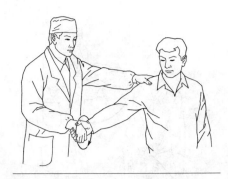

图149 握手摇肩
Fig. 149 Rotating of the shoulder while holding the hand

3. 抡摇肩关节

(以左肩关节为例)患者坐位，肩关节放松，自然下垂。操作者以丁字步站于其侧后方，以右手松握其腕背，左手手掌夹住其腕掌侧，慢慢向上举起(图150)；当上举到60°～120°范围时，托腕之左手反掌握住患者腕部，握腕之右手顺势向下滑移至肩关节上方按住；两手协调用力，右手按肩关节下压，左手握腕部上拉，使肩关节伸展，并继续将肩关节向上转动(图151)；当环转至240°～300°范围时，按肩之右手顺势滑移至腕部并握住，握腕之左手手指松开，以手掌夹住患者腕掌侧，并继续向下环转(图152)。连续操作3～5次后，再作自前向后环摇。操作者站于其侧前方，以左手松握其腕背，右手掌面夹住其腕掌侧，慢慢向前上方举起(图153)；当上举到60°～120°范围时，托腕之右手翻掌握住患者腕部，握腕之左手顺势向下滑移至肩部按住；两手协调用力，左手按肩关节下压，右手握腕部上拉，使肩关节伸展，并继续将肩关节向后转动(图154)；当环摇至240°～300°范围时，握肩之左手顺势滑回腕部并握住患者手腕，握腕之右手手指松开，以掌面夹住患者腕掌侧，并继续向前下环转(图155)。连续操作3～5次。本法适用于肩关节疼痛，关节活动功能障碍较轻患者。或经过推拿治疗，肩关节活动功能明显改善者。

3. Rotating of the shoulder like windmill

(Take left shoulder for example) The patient is in the

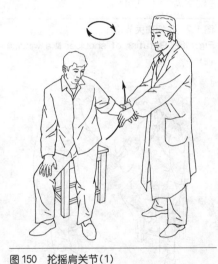

图150 抡摇肩关节(1)
Fig. 150 Rotating of shoulder like windmill (1)

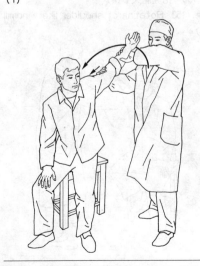

图151 抡摇肩关节(2)
Fig. 151 Rotating of shoulder like windmill (2)

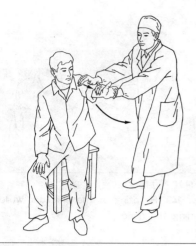

图 152 抡摇肩关节（3）
Fig. 152 Rotating of shoulder like windmill (3)

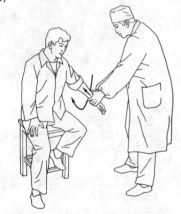

图 153 抡摇肩关节（4）
Fig. 153 Rotating of shoulder like windmill (4)

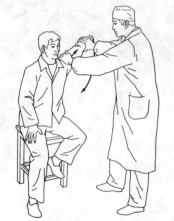

图 154 抡摇肩关节（5）
Fig. 154 Rotating of shoulder like windmill (5)

sitting position with his shoulder relaxed. The physician stands on the postero-laterior side with in the posture of forward lunge, loosely holds the wrist back with the right hand and clips the palm side of the wrist with the left palm. Then lifts the arm slowly(Fig.150). When the shoulder is being rotated in the range of 60° to 120°, the left hand which supported patient's wrist turns the palm and holds the wrist to continue lifting the arm up while the right hand moves along the arm to the superior side of the shoulder. With the two hands cooperating continually, the left hand drives the arm up and the right hand presses the shoulder down to stretch the shoulder and continue rotating (Fig.151). When the shoulder is being rotated in the range of 240° to 300°, the right hand which presses on the shoulder moves to the wrist and holds it while the left hand which holds the wrist loosens the fingers and clips the wrist. And then the two hands continues rotating shoulder downward (Fig.152). After repeating rotation for 3 to 5 circles, again rotates the shoulder anteriorly to posteriorly. The physician stands on the anterio-lateral side of the patient, loosely holds the wrist back with left hand, supports the palm side of the wrist with the right palm to lift the arm slowly directed anteriorly and superiorly(Fig.153). When the shoulder is being rotated in the range of 60° to 120°, the right hand which supports the wrist turns palm and continues holding the wrist, the left hand which holds the wrist loosens the fingers to move up along the arm to the shoulder. With the two hand coordinating, the left hand presses the shoulder down while the right hand holds the wrist to draw it upward so as to stretch the shoulder. Then continues rotating the shoulder backward (Fig.154). When the shoulder is being rotated in the range of 240° to 300°, the left hand moves along the arm to the wrist and holds it, the right hand loosens the fingers and supports the palm side of the wrist to rotate the shoulder(fig.155). The above rotation is repeated for 3 to 5 circles. This manipulation is suitable for those patients who have some troubles of shoulder pain, inconvenient motion of the shoulder or those patients whose motion function of the shoulder has been improved after Tuina therapy.

4. 卧位展筋摇肩

患者仰卧。操作者以弓步站于其患侧，一手按住患者三角肌部位，另一手握患者腕部，将患肢伸直上举至病理限制位；然后将患肢在维持轻度纵向牵引力下，以操作者的腰胯运动带动患者肩关节作小幅度环转运动(图156)。环转速度掌握在每分钟30～40次，顺时针方向、逆时针方向各作5～10次。本法适用于肩关节周围炎粘连期的治疗。

4. Rotating of the shoulder for stretching the tendon in supine position

The sufferer is in the supine position. The physician stands on the suffered side in the posture of forward lunge, and contacts the patient's deltoid with one hand and holds the wrist with the other hand. Then stretches and lifts the arm upward to the pathological limit position then drives the shoulder to be rotated in narrow range with the physician's lumbar and hip motion while the arm is being kept in slight traction(Fig.156). The speed of rotation is about 30 to 40 times per minute. The rotation is repeated for 5 to 10 circles at both clockwise and anticlockwise direction. This manipulation is adapted to cure the scapulohumeral periarthritis in the adhesion period.

5. 卧位点揉摇肩

患者仰卧。操作者以弓步站于患侧，用一手握住患者肘部将肩关节前屈至90°，另一手伸入肩胛骨下方，直到以手指触及肩胛骨内侧缘斜方肌、提肩胛肌、菱形肌附着处；边以指端点揉肩胛骨内侧缘，边带动肩关节作顺时针方向和逆时针方向环转摇动各10次；然后用指尖扣住肩胛骨内侧缘，与握患者肘部之手一同用力，将整个肩部向外侧拉伸至极限，再逐渐放松(图157)。本法适用于肩周炎粘连期治疗.

5. Rotating of the shoulder while kneading in supine position

The patient is in the supine position. The physician stands on the suffered side in the posture of forward lunge, holds the patient's elbow to flex the shoulder in 90° with one hand and touches the medial rim of the scapula where the trapezius, lavatory scapulae and rhomboid muscles are attached with the other hand fingers

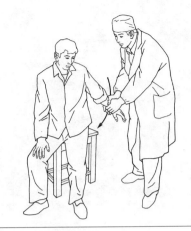

图155 抡摇肩关节(6)
Fig. 155 Rotating of shoulder like windmil1 (6)

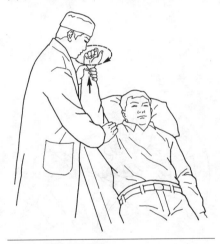

图156 卧位展筋摇肩
Fig. 156 Rotating of shoulder for stretching the tendon in supine position

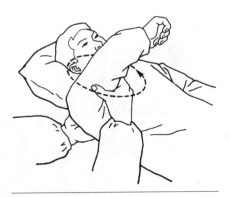

图157 卧位点揉摇肩
Fig. 157 Rotating of shoulder while kneading in supine position

which insert under the scapula. Then drives the shoulder to be rotated at the clockwise and anti-clockwise direction, while the fingers kneading the medial rim of the scapula. The shoulder is rotated for 10 circles at both directions. After that, the physician pulls the whole shoulder laterally to its limit with the finger tips of one hand hooking the medial rim of the scapula and the other hand holding the elbow, and then loosens it gradually(Fig.157). This manipulation is suitable for the treatment of scapulohumeral periarthritis in the adhesion period.

三、摇肘
Rotating of the Elbow

患者仰卧。操作者以弓步站于患侧，一手抓住其肘部，另一手抓住其腕部，作相对拔伸；然后在伸肘、轻度拔伸状态下利用操作者的躯体运动，带动肘关节作小幅度环转运动，顺时针、逆时针方向各10次；再在屈肘、轻度拔伸状态下，带动肘关节作环转运动(图158)。本法适用于肘关节疼痛、活动受限的治疗。

The patient is in the supine position. The physician stands on the suffered side in the posture of forward lunge, and holds the patient's elbow with one hand and the wrist with the other to pull the elbow oppositely. Then inducts the elbow to be rotated in narrow range with his trunk motion, while the suffered elbow is being in the extension and slightly traction. The rotation is repeated for 10 times at both clockwise and anti-clockwise direction. And then drives the elbow to do rotation in the flexion and slightly traction(Fig.158). This manipulation is suitable for the treatment of elbow pain with barricaded motion.

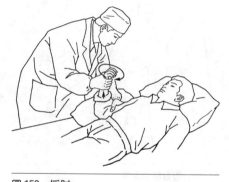

图158 摇肘

Fig. 158 Rotating of the elbow

四、摇腕
Rotating of the Wrist

患者坐位或仰卧位。操作者以一手握住患者前臂下端，另一手五指与患者手指相叉，作相对拔伸；然后在伸腕、轻度拔伸状态下带动腕关节作小幅度环转运动,顺时针与逆时针方向各5次。再在屈腕、轻度拔伸状态下带动腕关节作小幅度环转运动(图159)。本法适用于腕关节疼痛无力、活动障碍的治疗。

The patient is in the sitting position or supine position. The physician holds the lower end of the forearm with one hand and crosses the fingers with the fingers of the other hand to pull the wrist oppositely. Then inducts the wrist to be rotated in narrow range, while the suffered wrist is kept in the extension and slightly traction condition. The rotation is repeated for 5 times at both clockwise and anti-clockwise direction. And then drives the wrist to be rotated in the flexion and slightly traction condition(Fig. 159). This manipulation is suitable for the treatment of wrist pain with barricaded motion.

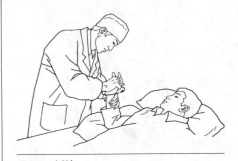

图159 摇腕
Fig. 159 Rotating of the wrist

五、摇指
Rotating of the Finger

患者坐位。操作者以一手握住患者手掌,另一手屈曲的示指和中指夹住患者手指,作相对拔伸;然后在维持拔伸状态下环摇掌指、指间关节(图160)。本法适用于指间、掌指关节疼痛肿胀、活动障碍的治疗。

The patient is in the sitting position. The physician holds the suffered palm with one hand and clips the suffered finger with the index and middle fingers of the other hand to pull the metacarpophalangeal joint or the interphalangeal joint oppositely. Then keeps the joint in traction and rotate the joint in narrow range(Fig.160). This manipulation is suitable for the treatment of pain, swollen and barricaded motion in the metacarpophalangeal joint or the interphalangeal joint.

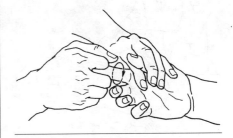

图160 摇指
Fig. 160 Rotating of the finger

六、摇腰
Rotating of the Lumbus

1. 坐位摇腰

患者坐位,腰部放松,略弯腰。操作者一手按住患者腰部,另一手扶持对侧肩部,两手协调,使腰部缓缓摇转。顺时针与逆时针方向各5～10次(图161)。本法适用于腰背酸痛、僵硬、活动不利的治疗。

1. Rotating of the lumbus in sitting position

The patient is in the sitting position, relaxes his lumbar muscles and flexes the lumbar slightly. The physician contacts the suffered side of the waist with one hand and supports the opposite shoulder with the other hand to rotate the lumbar slowly and coordinately. The rotation is repeated for 5 to 10 circles at both clockwise and anti-clockwise directions (Fig.161). This manipulation is suitable for the treatment of lower back pain, stiff lower back, and barricaded motion in lower back.

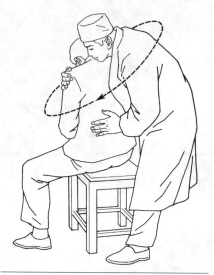

图161　坐位摇腰
Fig. 161　Rotating of the lumbus in sitting position

2. 卧位摇腰

患者仰卧位，屈膝屈髋。操作者以一手按于患者并拢之两膝部，另一手托住两小腿下端；然后带动患者两下肢作环转摇动，使患者骨盆与腰椎间亦产生环转运动，顺时针方向与逆时针方向各摇5～10次(图162)。本法适应证同上。

2. Rotating of the lumbus in supine position

The patient is in supine position, with his hip and knee joints flexed. The physician holds the two closed knees with one hand and supports the two lower ends of legs with the other hand. Then drives the two legs to be rotated, so that the pelvis and the lumbar intervertebral discs are also rotated slowly and coordinately. The rotation is repeated for 5 to 10 circles at both clockwise and anti-clockwise directions (Fig.162). The indication of this manipulation is same as the above one.

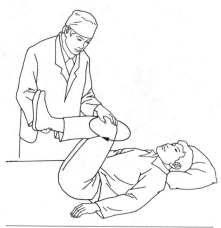

图162　卧位摇腰
Fig. 162　Rotating of the lumbus in supine position

七、摇髋
Rotating of the Hip

操作方式与卧位摇腰法相似，但仅环摇一侧下肢。由于一侧下肢伸直，骨盆处于稳定状态，故环转运动仅限于髋关节(图163)。本法适用于髋、股疼痛，活动不利的治疗。

The manipulative manner is like the above one, but only one leg is rotated. Because the other leg is in stretching condition and the pelvis in steady position, the rotation is localized in the hip joint (Fig. 163). This

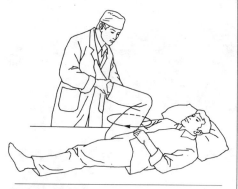

图163　摇髋
Fig. 163　Rotating of the hip

manipulation is suitable for the treatment of hip and thigh pain and barricaded motion of hip.

八、摇膝
Rotating of the Knee

患者仰卧位，膝关节半屈曲。操作者一手扶持其膝部，另一手握住其小腿下端；两手协调，使膝关节环转摇动，并边摇边慢慢将膝关节伸直，顺时针与逆时针方向各5～10次(图164)。本法适用于膝关节半月板破裂交锁状态的治疗。

The patient is in supine position, with his knee joints semi-flexed. The physician supports the knee with one hand and holds the end of leg with the other hand. Then drives the leg to be rotated slowly and coordinately, and then extends the knee while rotating. The rotation is repeated for 5 to 10 circles at both clockwise and anti-clockwise directions (Fig.164). This manipulation is suitable for the treatment of meniscus injury in lock condition.

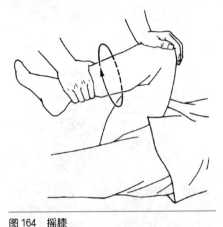

图 164 摇膝
Fig. 164 Rotating of the knee

九、摇踝
Rotating of the Ankle

患者仰卧位，下肢伸直。操作者一手托起其足跟，另一手握住其足前部，作纵向拔伸片刻；然后在维持轻度拔伸力下带动踝关节环转摇动(图165)。本法适用于踝关节扭伤、活动不利的治疗。

The patient is in supine position, with his leg stretched. The physician supports the heel with one hand and holds the forefoot with the other hand. Then hauls the ankle joint for a while. And then drives the ankle joint to be rotated while keeping in slight traction (Fig.165). This manipulation is suitable for the treatment of sprain of the ankle, as well as inconvenient motion of the ankle.

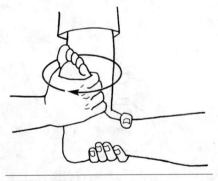

图 165 摇踝
Fig. 165 Rotating of the ankle

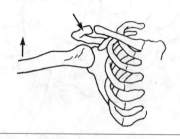

图166 推扳类手法模式图
Fig. 166 Model of category of the thrusting-wrenching manipulations

第十节 推扳类手法
SECTION 10 CATEGORY OF THE THRUSTING-WRENCHING MANIPULATIONS

所谓推扳类手法是指利用一对作用方向相反的力,使病变关节向某一特定方向作强制性运动,并突破该关节的病理或生理限制位,以达到分离粘连、正骨复位的目的的操作(图166)。由于这一类操作通常采用推或(和)扳两种动作所完成,故称之为推扳类手法。

The so-called category of the thrusting-wrenching manipulations means those actions in which one utilizes a double forces that are from opposite directions to drive the suffered joint to move to a special direction, so as to break the pathological or the physiological limitation of the joint and to reach the purposes of separating adhesion or restoring dislocation (Fig.166). Because these manipulations are usually completed by the motion of thrusting or wrenching, they are called as thrusting-wrenching manipulations.

一、扳颈
Wrenching of the Neck

1. 前屈展筋扳颈

患者仰卧。操作者站于其头端,两前臂十字交叉,托起患者枕部,两手则按住患者对侧肩部,组成一对省力杠杆;然后前臂抬起,带动患者颈椎缓缓前屈至极限位后复原,反复屈伸3～5次。本法能伸展痉挛的项后肌群与韧带,扩大颈椎后关节间隙,适用于颈项强硬,前屈不利者的治疗(图167)。

1. Flexion-wrenching of the neck for stretching the tendon

The patient is in the supine position. The physician stands on the rostral side, crosses the arms to support the patient's occiput, and contacts the opposite shoul-

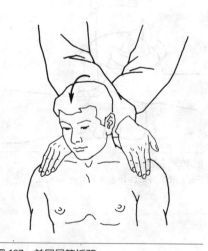

图167 前屈展筋扳颈
Fig. 167 Flexion-wrenching of the neck for stretching the tendon

ders of the patient with his hands to make up of a pair of levers that save labor. Then raises the forearm to drive the patient's cervical spine to be flexed to the limit position and then regains to original position. Repeats the motions as many as 3 to 5 times. This manipulation is able to stretch the convulsive muscles and tendons of the nape and expand the interval of the cervical facet joint. It is suitable for treating those who suffer from stiff neck and inconvenient flexion of the neck(Fig.167).

2. 侧屈展筋扳颈

患者坐位。操作者站于其偏后侧，以一手抱住患者头部并使之靠于胸前，另一手按住对侧肩部，两手协同用力，缓缓将患者颈椎侧屈至极限位后再复原，反复操作3~5次。本法能伸展痉挛的对侧颈肌和挛缩的韧带，并使对侧钩椎关节分离，适用于颈项疼痛僵硬、屈伸不利的治疗(图168)。

2. Lateral flexion-wrenching of the neck for stretching the tendon

The patient is in the sitting position. With standing on poster-lateral side, the physician holds the patient's head and keeps it against the chest with one hand, and contacts the opposite shoulder with the other hand. Then his two hands deliver force coordinately to make the patient's cervical spine laterally flexed to the limited position slowly, and then reverted to the neutral position. The above action is repeated for 3 to 5 times. This manipulation is able to stretch the convulsive cervical muscles and tendons of opposite side, and to cause the opposite Luschka's joint to be separated. It is suitable for the treatments of neck pain, stiff neck and inconvenient flexion and extension of the neck (Fig.168).

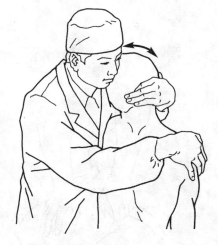

Fig.168 侧屈展筋扳颈
Fig. 168 Lateral flexion-wrenching of neck for stretching the tendon

3. 侧屈推扳法

患者坐位。操作者以一手拇指抵住偏凸之颈椎棘突，另一手按住患者对侧颞部，使其在略屈颈状态下侧屈至弹性限制位；然后两手协调用力，一手顶推颈椎棘突，另一手作一突发、有控制的侧向扳动，扩大颈椎侧屈幅度3°~5°，利用颈椎侧屈时伴随的旋转运动，使颈椎旋向对侧而复位(图169)。本法适用于中、下颈椎错缝的整复。

3. Lateral flexion-thrusting-wrenching of the neck

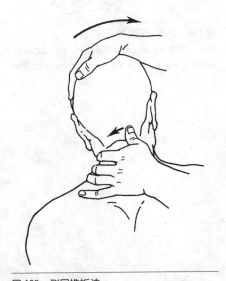

图169 侧屈推扳法
Fig. 169 Lateral flexion thrusting wrenching of the neck

The patient is in the sitting position. The physician contacts the projected spinous process of the suffered cervical vertebra with one thumb and the opposite temporal region with the other hand. Then makes the cervical spine laterally flexed to the elastic barrier under slight flexion of the neck. Then, while the thumb is resisting against the spinous process, the other hand makes a sudden and controlled lateral wrenching to expand the range of the lateral flexion in 3 to 5 degree, so as to utilize the rotation that is accompanied by the lateral flexion of the neck to cause restoration (Fig.169). This manipulation is adapted to the reduction of lower or middle cervical vertebral subluxation.

4. 卧位侧屈推扳法

患者俯卧，头旋向枢椎棘突偏凸侧。操作者站于其前面，以一手按住患者颞部固定之，另一手拇指按压枢椎棘突的上面，余四指提扣颈2及以下颈椎棘突的下面；然后上提颈椎使之向下侧屈至弹性限制位，随后作一突发有控制的上提动作，扩大颈椎侧屈幅度3°～5°，同时拇指向下顶推，四指向上扳扣，使颈椎复位（图170）。本法适用于寰枢椎错缝整复，也可用于颈4以上的椎骨错缝复位。

4. Lateral flexion-thrusting-wrenching of the neck in prone position

The patient is in the prone position, with his head rotated toward the side on which the suffered spinous process of the C2 is projected. Standing in front of the patient, the physician contacts the temporal region to fix the head with a hand, and spinous process of the C2 with the other hand, with the thumb put on spinous process of the C2 and the rest finger under that of the lower cervical vertebrae. Then pulls the spinous processes of the lower cervical vertebrae upward, so that the cervical spine is laterally flexed to the elastic barrier position. Then makes a sudden and controlled wrenching to expand the lateral flexion range in 3 to 5 degree. At the same time, thrusts the spinous process of the C2 downward with the thumb and wrenches that of the rest fingers upward to turn the two vertebrae of the same motion segment oppositely. In this way, the subluxation

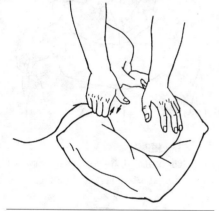

图170　卧位侧屈推扳法
Fig. 170 Lateral flexion thrusting-wrenching of the neck in prone position

is usually reverted to their anatomical relation (Fig.170). This manipulation is adapted to the reduction of C1, C2 vertebral subluxation or those subluxation that are above the C4.

5. 卧位侧屈牵引扳

患者仰卧。操作者站于其头端，两手虎口分开，拇指向上，扣住患者下颌骨；余手指向下，环抱患者枕部，作颈椎纵向牵引片刻。然后在维持轻度牵引力下将颈椎向其棘突偏凸侧侧屈至弹性限制位；侧屈时注意保持患者头部冠状面处于水平位置，再作一突发而有控制的动作，微屈颈椎5°～10°，使错缝关节受到震动而复位(图171)。本法适用于下颈椎椎骨错缝的整复。

5. Lateral flexion-wrenching of the neck under traction in supine position

The patient is in the supine position. The physician stands on the rostral side, opens the first web of hands, keeps the thumbs upward and the rest fingers downward to hold the patient's chin and the occiput. Then pulls the cervical spine for a while, and then laterally flexes the neck toward the suffered side to its elastic barrier position. While keeping in slight traction. It would be noted to keep the frontal plane of the head in horizontal line during lateral flexion. Latter, makes a sudden and controlled action to flex the cervical spine in 5 to 10 degree, so that the subluxation segment is shocked and restored (Fig.171). This manipulation is adapted to the reduction of lower cervical subluxation.

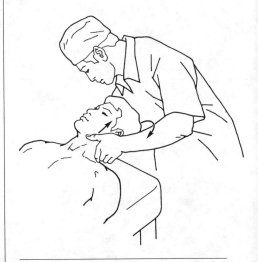

图171 卧位侧屈牵引扳

Fig. 171 Lateral flexion-wrenching of the neck under traction in supine position

6. 坐位斜扳法

患者坐位，微屈颈，放松颈部肌肉。操作者以一手托患者下颌，另一手托患者枕部，使头颈向旋转运动受限侧旋转至弹性限制位，然后作一突发有控制扳动，扩大旋转幅度3°～5°。本法可充分伸展斜方肌上部及胸锁乳突肌，整复上颈椎错缝。但由于操作时定位性差，对下颈椎错缝有造成颈部损伤的可能性(图172)。

6. Oblique-wrenching of the neck in sitting position

The patient is in the sitting position, slightly flexes the neck to relax the cervical muscles. The physician supports the patient's chin with one hand and the occiput

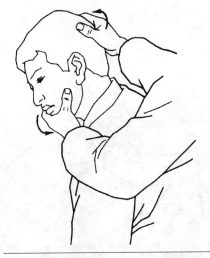

图172 坐位斜扳法

Fig. 172 Oblique-wrenching of the neck in sitting position

with the other hand to inducts the head rotated toward the side on which the neck rotation is limited to its elastic barrier position. Then makes a sudden and controlled wrenching to expand the rotation range in 3 to 5 degree. This manipulation can fully stretch the upper portion of the muscle trapezium and sternocleidomastoid, restore upper cervical vertebral subluxation. But due to its inability to select acting level accurately, it will be possible to cause injury of neck, if this manipulation is used to restore lower cervical vertebral subluxation (Fig.172).

7. 卧位斜扳法

患者仰卧。操作者以双手环托患者下颌及颞枕部，在保持颈椎轻度前屈位下将头向后上方牵引片刻，然后在维持牵引力下将患者头部旋转向棘突偏凸侧，至弹性限制位后再作一突发有控制扳动，扩大旋转幅度3°～5°，即可复位(图173)。本法适用于中上颈段椎骨错缝的整复。

7. Oblique-wrenching of the neck in supine position

The patient is in the supine position. The physician holds his chin and occiput to pull directed posterior superior for a while with hands. Then while keeping in traction, makes the patient's head rotated toward the side on which the suffered spinous process is projected. After reaching its elastic barrier position, a sudden and controlled action is done to expand the rotation range in 3 to 5 degree. Thus the facet joint is restored(Fig.173). This manipulation is adapted to the reduction of middle and upper cervical vertebral subluxation.

8. 卧位侧屈旋转扳

患者仰卧。操作者双手抱住其下颌及颞枕部向后上牵拉，在牵引状态下将患者颈椎侧屈及使头部向对侧旋转约45°，至弹性限制位后，作一突发有控制动作，将头部自上而下扳抖，使颈椎复位。本法适用于颈椎错缝伴颈椎生理前凸平直患者的整复，但对颈椎生理前凸增加的患者有引起椎动脉损伤的可能，应慎用(图174)。

8. Lateral flexion-rotation-wrenching of the neck in supine position

The patient is in the supine position. The physician holds the chin and occiput to pull directed posterior

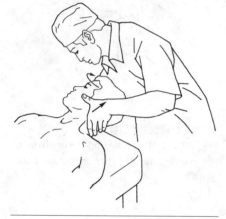

图173 卧位斜扳法
Fig. 173 Oblique-wrenching of the neck in supine position

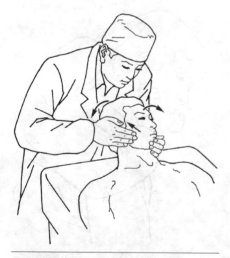

图174 卧位侧屈旋转扳
Fig. 174 Lateral flexion-rotation-wrenching of the neck in supine position

superiorly with hands. In this way, the patient's head is laterally flexed and oppositely rotated about 45 degree under traction. After the neck reaching its elastic barrier position, the physician makes a sudden and controlled action to shake the head from superior to inferior to cause the cervical vertebrae restoration. This manipulation is suitable for those sufferers whose subluxation is accompanied with flattened cervical curvature. But for those accompanied with cervical lordosis, applying this manipulation may cause the injury of vertebral arteries. So one must keep in heart that it should be used carefully (Fig. 174).

9. 坐位摇扳法

患者坐位，两下肢前伸，略弯腰弓背屈颈，使竖脊肌完全放松。操作者一手托住患者下颌、面颊，另一手拇指顶推偏凸之棘突。然后使患者头颈作小幅度环摇动作，并不断调整颈椎屈伸幅度，直至找到恰当的位置。此时操作者拇指感到项肌放松，另一手摇颈时亦无阻力；再在摇颈基础上将颈推向棘突偏凸侧扳动，突破弹性限制位3°～5°，即可复位。本法适用于中上颈椎错缝的整复(图175)。

9. Rotating-wrenching of the neck in sitting position

The patient is in the sitting position, with his low limbs stretched forward and the spine flexed slightly so as to fully relax the erector spinal muscles. The physician holds the patient's chin and cheek with one hand, contacts against the projected spinous process with the thumb of the other hand. Then rotates the patient's head in narrow range and adjusts the flexion-extension position of the neck step by step, until a suitable posture to be found. In this posture, the physician can feel the nape muscles being fully relaxed and the spinous process moved as his rotation action under the thumb. At the very time when the head is rotated to its elastic barrier position of the suffered side, wrenches the head and thrusts the spinous process simultaneously to expand the rotation range in 3 to 5 degree. Thus the facet joint may be restored. This manipulation is adapted to the reduction of the middle and upper cervical vertebrae subluxation (Fig. 175).

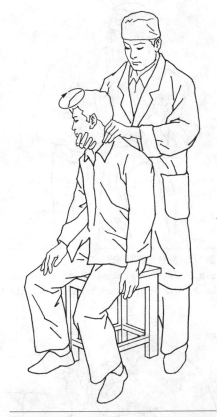

图175 坐位摇扳法
Fig.175 Rotating-wrenching of the neck in sitting position

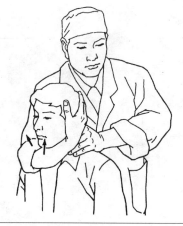

图176 旋转定位扳前视
Fig. 176 Frontal view of rotation-wrenching of the neck on selected site

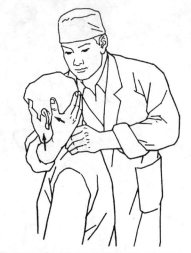

图177 旋转定位扳侧视
Fig. 177 Lateral view of rotation wrenching of the neck on selected site

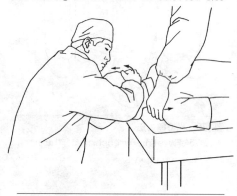

图178 俯卧位牵引旋转扳
Fig. 178 Rotation-wrenching of the neck under traction in prone position

10. 旋转定位扳法

患者坐位。操作者以一手屈曲之肘部托住患者下颌，手指托住枕部，另一手拇指顶推偏凸之颈椎棘突；令患者逐渐屈颈，至拇指感觉偏凸棘突之上间隙开始分离，即维持该屈颈幅度；然后操作者将患者头部向上牵拉片刻，以克服颈肌反射性收缩，再逐渐将颈部向棘突偏凸旋转侧旋转至弹性限制位，作一突发有控制的扳动，扩大旋转幅度3°～5°，同时拇指用力顶推棘突，使颈椎复位(图176，177)。本法适用于全颈椎椎骨错缝。

10. Rotation-wrenching of the neck on selected site

The patient is in the sitting position. The physician supports the patient's chin with his flexed elbow and holds the occiput with one hand, contacts against projected spinal process of the suffered segment with the thumb of other hand. Then guides the patient to flex neck gradually. When the thumb feels the above interval of spinous process is broadened, stops flexion and keeps the neck in this position. Then pulls the head upward for a while to get rid of the reflective contraction of the muscles. Latter, rotates the neck toward the side, on which the spinous process of the suffered segment is projected to its elastic barrier position. Makes a sudden and controlled wrenching to expand the rotation range in 3 to 5 degree. At the same time, the thumb thrusts the spinous process to cause the facet joint to be restored(Fig. 176, 177). This manipulation is adapted to all the cervical vertebral subluxation.

11. 俯卧位牵引旋转扳

患者俯卧，头颈伸出床沿。助手两手按住其双肩及颈根部，使错位节段以下颈椎保持稳定。操作者坐于患者头前，两手十指相扣，肘关节屈曲，以双手及前臂环抱患者头部；嘱患者放松，在颈轻度前屈位下牵伸患者颈椎片刻，待患者反射性肌痉挛消除后，先将头颈向棘突偏凸侧旋转至弹性限制位，作一突发轻巧扳动，扩大旋转幅度3°～5°，随即放松；再将颈椎反向旋转至弹性限制位，作一突发轻巧扳动，即可复位(图178)。本法适用于所有颈椎椎骨错缝的整复。

11. Rotation-wrenching of the neck under traction in prone position

The patient is in the prone position, with his neck

stretched out of the bed end. An assistant holds the shoulders and the neck bottom to keep the cervical vertebrae in steady. The physician sits in front of the patient's head, crosses his fingers of the two hands and flexes the elbow to hold the head around with his hands and forearms. Then guides the patient to be relaxed, and pulls the cervical spine for a while in slight flexion position. When the patient's reflection spasm of muscle has been relieved, rotates the neck toward the side, where the spinous process is projected to its elastic barrier position at first. Then makes a sudden and controlled wrenching to expand the rotation range in 3 to 5 degree and then loosens the neck immediately. When the manipulation is repeated at the contralateral direction, the subluxation can be restored(Fig.178). This manipulation is adapted to the reduction of all the cervical vertebral subluxation.

[附] 滚法与颈项扳法配合操作
[Appendix] Operation of Rolling Coordinated with Wrenching of Neck

患者坐位。操作者先以滚法在患者颈项及肩背部操作,滚患者左侧颈项肩背时宜用右手,而滚右侧时则采用左手,以方便操作。在颈项肩背部充分使用滚法,患者局部疼痛及肌紧张均有缓解的基础上,配合颈项扳法。操作者一手扶持患者额部,另一手继续在颈项部操作;当滚到枕下部位时,扶额部之手使患者屈颈至疼痛限制位,并作一突发有控制扳动,扩大前屈幅度3°～5°(图179);当滚到颈根部时,扶额部之手使患者颈部后伸至疼痛限制位并作一突发有控制扳动,扩大后伸幅度3°～5°(图180);当滚左侧颈肩部时,扶额部之手使患者颈部向左旋转至疼痛限制位,并作一突发有控制扳动,扩大左旋幅度3°～5°(图181);当滚右侧颈肩部时,扶额部之手使患者颈部向右旋转至疼痛限制位,并作突发有控制的扳动,扩大右旋幅度3°～5°(图181)。以上操作方式,各重复2～3次。随后操作者以一手扶持患者额部,用与患侧同侧之手在颈外侧施以滚法,逐渐将患者颈部向对侧侧屈至疼痛限制位,并作一突发有控制的扳动,扩大侧屈幅度3°～5°,重复以上操作2～3次,再在对侧作相同操作(图182)。本法适用于落枕、颈椎病、颈部软组织劳损等病症的治疗。

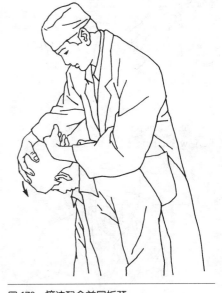

图179 滚法配合前屈扳颈
Fig. 179 Rolling coordinated with flexion-wrenching of the neck

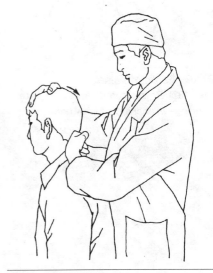

图180 滚法配合后伸扳颈
Fig. 180 Rolling coordinated with extension-wrenching of the neck

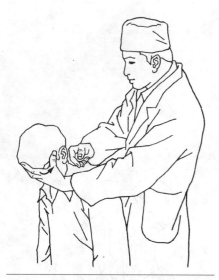

图181 滚法配合旋转扳颈
Fig. 181 Rolling coordinated with rotation-wrenching of the neck

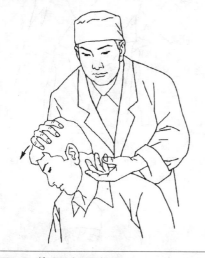

图182 滚法配合侧屈扳颈
Fig. 182 Rolling coordinated with lateral bending-wrenching of the neck

The patient is in the sitting position. The physician manipulates on the patient's nape, shoulder and back regions with rolling. The right hand should be used for rolling on the left side, and the left hand be used for rolling on the right side, so as to make the manipulation easier. When the acted regions have received full stimulus of the rolling and local pain and muscle contraction have been relieved. wrenching can be cooperated. During this stage, one hand supports the patient's forehead, while the other hand continues rolling on the nape region. When the hand is rolling on the occiput region, the hand which supports the forehead leads the neck to be flexed to its painful barrier position and makes a sudden, controlled wrenching to expand the flexion range in 3 to 5 degree (Fig.179). When the hand is rolling on the bottom of neck, the other hand drives the neck to be extended to its painful barrier position and makes a sudden and controlled wrenching to expand extension range in 3 to 5 degree (Fig.180). If rolling on the left side, the homolateral hand rotates the neck leftward to its painful barrier position and makes a sudden and controlled wrenching to expand rotation range in 3 to 5 degree (Fig.181). If rolling on right side, the right hand rotates the neck rightward to its painful barrier position and makes a sudden and controlled wrenching to expand rotation range in 3 to 5 degree(Fig.181). Repeats the above actions for 2 to 3 times. Then the physician holds the temple region with one hand, delivers rolling on the lateral region of the neck with the homolateral hand. Laterally bends the neck at opposite direction gradually to its painful barrier position, and makes a sudden and controlled wrenching to expand lateral bending range in 3 to 5 degree. Repeats this action for 2 to 3 times. Again repeats the same action on the opposite side (Fig.182). These manipulations are adapted to the treatments of neck sprain, cervical spondylopathy and the strain of soft tissues of neck.

二、扳肩
Wrenching of the Shoulder

1. 前举扳肩
患者坐位。操作者半蹲于其侧前方，将患者伸直之上肢搁置于自己肩上，两手手指交叉后按住患者肩部；然后下肢逐渐伸直，把患者肩关节上举至弹性限制位，再作一突发有控制扳动，扩大上举幅度3°～5°，随即放松(图183)。重复操作3～5次。本法适用于肩关节周围炎粘连期上举活动障碍的治疗。

1. Flexion-wrenching of the shoulder
The patient is in the sitting position. With standing in semi-squat posture on the latero-anterior side, the physician puts the patient's stretched upper limb on his shoulder, and presses the patient's shoulder with his crossed fingers. Then stretches his lower limbs to raise the patient's arm step by step to its elastic barrier position and makes a sudden and controlled wrenching to expand the flexion range in 3 to 5 degree, and loosens at once (Fig.183). Repeats the action for 3 to 5 times. This manipulation is adapted to the treatment of flexion obstruction of the scapulohumeral periarthritis in the adhesion period.

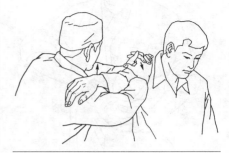

图 183 前举扳肩
Fig. 183 Flexion-wrenching of the shoulder

2. 外展扳肩
操作方式基本同前举扳肩，但操作者站于患者外侧，将肩关节外展扳举(图184)。本法适用于肩周炎粘连期外展运动障碍的治疗。

2. Abduction-wrenching of the shoulder
The manipulative manner is very similar to the above. But the physician stands on the lateral side and wrenches the shoulder at abducent direction(Fig.184). This manipulation is adapted to the treatment of abducent obstruction of scapulohumeral periarthritis in the adhesion period.

3. 内收扳肩
患者坐位，患侧之手放于胸前。操作者站于其身后，以胸部紧靠其背，稳定躯干；以与患肩对侧之手从其对侧肩上伸过，握住患腕；与患肩同侧之手则从患肩外侧伸过，胳膊包绕肩部，用手托住患肘；然后两手协同，握腕之手向后拉，托肘

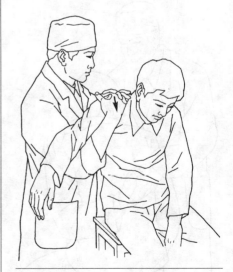

图 184 外展扳肩
Fig. 184 Abduction-wrenching of the shoulder

之手向内侧推,至内收限制位后,作一突发有控制的扳动,扩大内收幅度3°～5°,随即放松。重复操作3~5次(图185)。本法适用于肩周炎粘连期内收运动障碍的治疗。

3. Adduction-wrenching of the shoulder

The patient is in the sitting position, puts the hand of the suffered side in front of the chest. With standing behind the patient, The physician leans his chest against the patient's back to steady the patient's trunk, holds patient's wrist of suffered side with his contralateral hand, stretches the homolateral hand to hold the patient's elbow with the arm that is around the suffered shoulder. Then uses the hand that holds the wrist to pull backward while the hand that holds the elbow to push medially to the adductive barrier position. With the two hands acting coordinately, makes a sudden and controlled wrenching-thrusting to expand the adduction range in 3 to 5 degree. Loosens the shoulder at once. Repeats this manipulation for 3 to 5 times (Fig.185). This manipulation is adapted to the treatment of the adductive obstruction of the scapulohumeral periarthritis in the adhesion period.

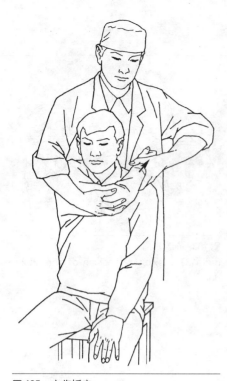

图185 内收扳肩
Fig. 185 Adduction-wrenching of the shoulder

4. 后弯扳肩

患者坐位。操作者站于其侧后方,一手按于患肩,稳定关节,另一手握住患腕,并逐渐将其肩关节后伸内旋屈肘至极限位,手背紧贴背部;然后作一突发有控制的扳动,使患手沿背脊向上滑移半个棘突高度,随即迅速放松(图186)。重复操作3~5次。本法适用于肩周炎粘连期后弯(摸背)运动障碍的治疗。

4. Posterior bending-wrenching of the shoulder

The patient is in the sitting position. The physician stands on the laterio-posterior side of him, presses the suffered shoulder to steady it with one hand, holds the wrist of suffered side to make the upper limb in such position, in which the shoulder is extended and rotated, the elbow is flexed and the back of hand is kept close to patient's back with the other hand. Then makes a sudden and controlled wrenching to move the patient's hand upward for half width of a spinous process along the back. Loosens immediately (Fig.186). Repeats these ac-

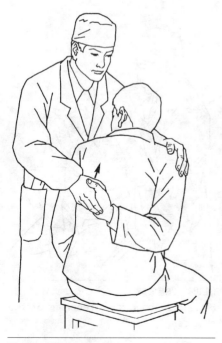

图186 后弯扳肩
Fig. 186 Posterior bending-wrenching of the shoulder

tions for 3 to 5 times. This manipulation is adapted to the treatment of posterior bending obstruction of the scapulohumeral periarthritis in the adhesion period.

5. 旋转扳肩

患者坐位。操作者站于其侧后方，以一足踏于凳上，膝盖顶住腋窝；一手按于患肩，稳定关节，另一手握住患肢前臂上端，慢慢将肩关节外展至90°（或外展至限制位），然后将肩关节逐渐外旋至极限位，作一突发有控制运动，扩大外旋幅度3°～5°，随即放松（图187）；再逐渐将肩关节内旋至极限位，作一突发有控制扳动，扩大内旋幅度3°～5°，随即放松。重复操作3～5次。本法适用于肩周炎粘连期旋转运动障碍的治疗。

5. Rotation-wrenching of the shoulder

The patient is in the sitting position. The physician stands behind him, with a foot stepping on the chair and the knee resisting against the patient's armpit. Presses on the suffered shoulder with one hand to steady the joint, holds the upper part of the forearm with the other hand and keeps the shoulder abducted to 90 degree (If 90° can't be reached, the shoulder may be abducted to its barrier position). Then rotates the shoulder lateriorly to its barrier position, and makes a sudden and controlled wrenching to expand the range of the laterior rotation in 3 to 5 degree, loosens it immediately (Fig. 187). Latter, medially rotates the shoulder gradually to its barrier position and makes a sudden and controlled wrenching to expand the range of the medial rotation in 3 to 5 degree and loosens it immediately. Repeats these actions for 3 to 5 times. These manipulations are adapted to the treatment of the rotative obstruction of the scapulohumeral periarthritis in the adhesion period.

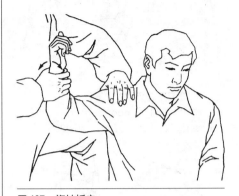

图187　旋转扳肩
Fig. 187　Rotation-wrenching of the shoulder

[附] 滚法与肩关节扳法配合操作
[Appendix] Manipulations of Rolling Coordinated with Wrenching of the Shoulder

1. 坐位操作

患者坐位。操作者先在患侧肩颈背部作滚法操作，待该部位经过充分滚法刺激，在局部疼痛和肌紧张已初步缓解的基础

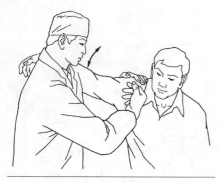

图188 滚法配合外展扳肩
Fig. 188 Rolling coordinated with abduction wrenching of the shoulder

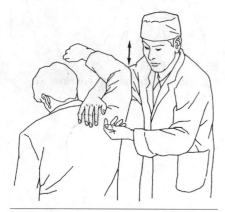

图189 滚法配合前屈扳肩
Fig. 189 Rolling coordinated with flexion wrenching of the shoulder

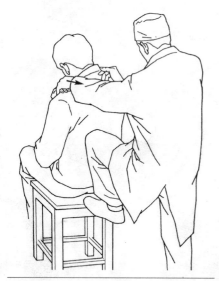

图190 滚法配合内收扳肩
Fig. 190 Rolling coordinated with adduction wrenching of the shoulder

上，配合肩关节各方向的扳法。操作者先以与患侧同侧之手继续在肩前部进行滚法刺激，另一手从患肩腋下穿过，自肩后方按住肩关节，使之稳定；边滚边将患肢外展至疼痛限制位，并作一突发有控制扳动，扩大外展幅度3°～5°，随即放松（图188），重复以上操作3～5遍。接着操作者交换双手，以与患侧对侧之手在肩后部继续进行滚法刺激，另一手从患肩腋下穿过，自肩前方按住肩关节，使之稳定；边滚边将患肢前举至疼痛限制位，并作一突发有控制扳动，扩大前举幅度3°～5°，随即放松（图189），重复以上操作3～5遍。随后操作者站于患者背后，以与患肩对侧之膝部顶住患者后背，对侧手则从患者对侧肩上伸过，握住患者放在胸前之患手并向后拉至疼痛限制位，与患者同侧之手则继续在患肩外侧进行滚法刺激，边滚边配合突发有控制的内收扳动，超过内收限制位3°～5°，随即放松（图190），重复以上操作3～5次。再以一侧膝盖顶入患肩腋下，足尖则踏于凳沿上，使患肩处于外展位置，肘部屈曲，用一手握住其上臂下端，另一手在肩前部进行滚法操作，边滚边将肩关节外旋至疼痛限制位，并作一突发轻巧的扳动，扩大外旋幅度3°～5°，随即放松（图191），重复以上操作3～5次。交换一下左右手，以原握臂之手在肩后方进行滚法操作，原滚法操作之手则握住上臂下端，边滚边将肩关节内旋至疼痛极限位，并作一突发轻巧的扳动，扩大内旋幅度3°～5°，随即放松，重复以上操作3～5次。最后作滚法与后弯扳肩的配合，操作者以一手握患手使其肩关节后伸、内旋，肘关节屈曲，手背沿脊背上移至疼痛限制位，另一手继续在肩关节前方进行按法刺激，边滚边配合后弯扳动，作一突发、轻巧的扳动，使患者手背紧贴后背向上移动半个棘突高度，随即放松（图192），重复以上操作3～5次。

1. Manipulation in sitting position

The patient is in sitting position. The physician exerts the rolling manipulation on the nape, shoulder and back regions of the suffered side at first. After these regions have received full stimulus of rolling and the local pain and the muscle contraction have been relieved, the rolling should be coordinated with the wrenching in all directions. The physician continually exerts rolling stimulus on the anterior region of the shoulder with the homolateral hand, puts the contralateral hand that is passed through the armpit on the shoulder to steady it. Then inducts the shoulder to be abducted to its painful barrier position and makes a sudden and controlled wrenching to expand the abduction range in 3 to 5 degree while rolling. Loosens immediately(Fig.188). Repeats the action for 3 to 5 times. Then the physician exchanges his two hands work, delivers the rolling to stimulate the posterior region of the shoulder with the hand that is contralateral to the patient and presses the shoulder from front of the shoulder with the other hand that goes through the armpit to steady it. Drives the shoulder to be flexed to its painful barrier position and makes a sudden and controlled wrenching to expand the flexion range in 3 to 5 degree.Loosens it immediately (Fig.189).Repeats the above action for 3 to 5 times. Latter, the physician stands behind the patient,resists against the patient's back with his knee that is contralateral to the suffered shoulder, holds the hand of suffered side, which is put in the front of the chest, and pulls it backward to the painful barrier position with the hand that is stretched over the patient's opposite shoulder, exerts rolling stimulus continually on the laterior portion of the shoulder with the other hand. Coordinates with sudden and controlled thrusting to adduct the shoulder to surpass its adductive barrier position in 3 to 5 degree, while rolling.Loosens the shoulder immediately(Fig.190). Repeats the above action for 3 to 5 times. Next, supports the armpit with a flexed knee, while the tiptoe is stepping on the chair, makes the suffered shoulder in abduction and the elbow in flexion. Holds the lower end of the upper arm with one hand, exerts the rolling on the anterior region of the shoulder with the other hand.After that, rotates the shoulder to its painful barrier position and wrenches it suddenly and gently to expand lateral rotation range in 3 to 5 degree. Loosens the shoulder immediately(Fig.191). Repeats the above action for 3 to 5 times.Then exchanges the hands to deliver rolling on the posterior region of the shoulder with the hand that holds the arm formerly and holds the lower portion of the arm with the other hand to rotates the shoulder medially to its painful barrier position. And then wrenches it suddenly and gently to expand medial rotation range in 3 to 5 degree.Loosens the shoulder immediately. Repeats the above action for 3 to 5 times.

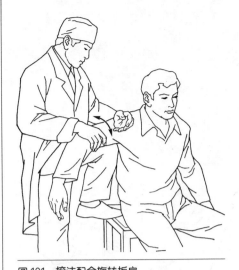

Fig. 191 Rolling coordinated with rotation wrenching of the shoulder

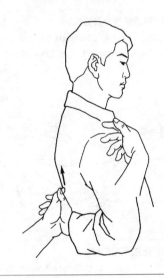

Fig. 192 Rolling coordinated with posterior bending wrenching of the shoulder

Finally, coordinates rolling with posterior bending-wrenching of the shoulder. The physician holds the homolateral hand to cause the shoulder joint to be extended posterior and rotate medially, the elbow joint to be flexed and the hand back to be kept close to the back of the patient. Pulls the handback suddenly and gently to move upward along the back for half height of a spinous process and loosens the shoulder immediately, while rolling (Fig.192). Repeats the above action for 3 to 5 times.

2. 卧位操作

患者仰卧。操作者站于患侧，一手继续在肩前部施以㨰法操作，另一手托起患者上臂下端，使其肩关节外展，并将其肘部靠于操作者腰部；边㨰边用躯体运动将肩关节外展至疼痛限制位，作一突发有控制扳动，扩大外展幅度3°～5°，随即放松，重复以上操作3～5次(图193)。接着令患者侧卧，操作者站于其前面，一手继续在肩关节后方进行㨰法刺激，另一手托住上臂下端，并将其肘部靠于操作者腰部，边㨰边用躯体运动将患者肩关节前举至疼痛限制位，并作突发有控制的扳动，扩大肩关节前举幅度3°～5°随即放松，重复以上操作3～5次(图194)。然后令患者屈肘，一手托住患者肘后，另一手继续在肩关节外侧施以㨰法，边㨰边将肩关节内收至疼痛限制位，并作一突发有控制扳动，扩大内收幅度3°～5°，随即放松(图195)，重复以上操作3～5次。再以一手握住患者上臂下端，使其肩关节外展，另一手继续在腋窝处施以㨰法，边㨰边将肩关节外展至疼痛限制位，作一突发有控制的扳动，扩大外展幅度3°～5°，随即放松(图196)。重复以上操作3～5次。随后令患者仰卧，操作者站于其头侧，以一手在肩关节前方施以㨰法，另一手握住其上臂下端逐渐上举至疼痛限制位，作一突发轻巧扳动，扩大前举幅度3°～5°，随即放松，重复以上操作3～5次(图197)。患者体位不变，操作者站于患侧，以一手在肩关节前方施以㨰法，另一手握住其前臂下端，将其屈肘，肩关节外展；边㨰边将肩关节外旋至疼痛限制位，作一突发轻巧扳动，扩大外旋幅度3°～5°，随即放松，重复以上操作3～5次(图198)。最后令患者侧卧，操作者一手握住患者腕部将其肩关节后伸、内旋，肘关节屈曲，仿摸背动作，另一手继续在肩前方施㨰法，边㨰边将其患手沿脊背后上拉至疼痛限制位，作一突发有控制扳动，提高摸背高度半个棘突。随即放松。重复以上操作3～5次。

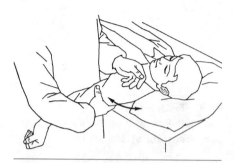

图193　㨰法配合外展扳肩
Fig. 193 Rolling coordinated with abduction wrenching of the shoulder

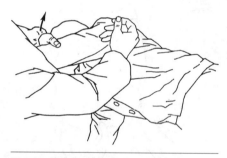

图194　㨰法配合前屈扳肩
Fig. 194 Rolling coordinated with flexion wrenching of the shoulder

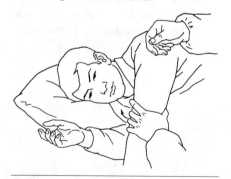

图195　㨰法配合内收扳肩
Fig. 195 Rolling coordinated with adduction wrenching of the shoulder

2. Manipulation in lying position

The patient lies in the supine position. The physician stands on the suffered side, delivers rolling on the anterior portion of the shoulder with one hand, supports the lower portion of the upper arm to keep the shoulder in abduction and the elbow in leaning against his waist. Then takes the advantage of the trunk motion to abduct the shoulder to its painful barrier position and makes a sudden and controlled motion to expand abduction range in 3 to 5 degree, while rolling. Loosens the shoulder immediately. Repeats the above action for 3 to 5 times (Fig.193). After that, guides the patient in side lying position. The physician stands in front of the patient, delivers rolling stimulus on the posterior region of the shoulder with one hand, supports the lower portion of the upper arm with the other hand and puts the elbow against the waist. Then takes advantage of the trunk movement to flex the shoulder to its painful barrier position, and makes a sudden and controlled wrenching to expand flexion range in 3 to 5 degree. Loosens the shoulder immediately. Repeats the above action for 3 to 5 times(Fig.194). Then asks the patient to flex his elbow. Supports the elbow with one hand, delivers rolling on the lateral portion of the shoulder with the other hand. Then drives the shoulder to be adducted to its painful barrier position, and makes a sudden and controlled wrenching to expand adductive range in 3 to 5 degree. Loosens the shoulder immediately (Fig.195). Repeats the above action for 3 to 5 times. Again holds the lower end of the upper arm with one hand to abduct the shoulder, delivers rolling on the armpit with other hand, inducts the shoulder to be abducted to its painful barrier position and makes a sudden and controlled wrenching to expand abducent range in 3 to 5 degree. Loosens the shoulder immediately(Fig.196). Repeats the above action for 3 to 5 times. Latter, guides the patient to lie in the supine position. The physician stands on the rostral side, delivers rolling on the anterior portion of the shoulder with one hand, holds the lower portion of the upper arm with the other hand to flex the shoulder to painful barrier position gradually, then makes a sudden and gentle wrenching to

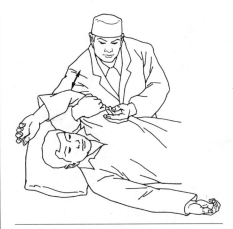

Fig. 196 Rolling on armpit coordinated with abduction wrenching of the shoulder

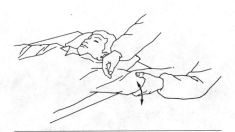

Fig. 197 Rolling coordinated with flexion wrenching of the shoulder

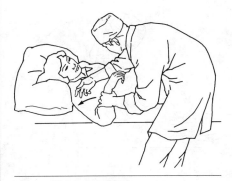

Fig. 198 Rolling coordinated with lateral rotation wrenching of the shoulder

expand flexion range in 3 to 5 degree. Loosens the shoulder immediately. Repeats the above actions for 3 to 5 times (Fig.197). The patient's posture is kept in the same as the above step. The physician stands on the suffered side, delivers rolling on the anterior region of the shoulder with one hand, holds the lower end of the forearm with the other hand to keep the elbow in flexion and the shoulder in abduction. Laterally rotates the shoulder to painful barrier position and makes a sudden and gentle wrenching to expand lateral rotation range in 3 to 5 degree, while rolling. Loosens the shoulder immediately. Repeats the above action for 3 to 5 times (Fig. 198). Finally, asks the patient to lie in side position. The physician holds the wrist of suffered side to make the shoulder joint be extended posteriorly, rotated medially and the elbow joint flexed as the motion of touching back. While the other hand continually rolls on the anterior region of the shoulder, pulls the hand upward along the back to painful barrier position and makes a sudden and controlled wrenching to increase the height of touching back for half width of a spinous process, while rolling. Repeats the above action for 3 to 5 times.

三、扳肘
Wrenching of the Elbow

1. 屈曲扳肘

患者仰卧，操作者以一手托患肘后方，另一手握住前臂下端，逐渐将肘关节屈曲至疼痛限制位，然后作一突发有控制扳动，扩大肘屈曲幅度3°～5°（图199）。本法可紧张肘关节囊后壁，挤破肘关节血肿，使之流入肱三头肌间隙，以利吸收。适用于肘关节血肿、肘关节屈曲功能障碍的治疗。

1. Flexion-wrenching of the elbow

The patient is in the supine position. The physician supports the posterior region of the elbow with one hand, holds the lower end of the forearm with the other hand. The elbow is flexed gradually to painful barrier position. Then a sudden and controlled wrenching is done to expand the flexion range in 3 to 5 degree (Fig.199).

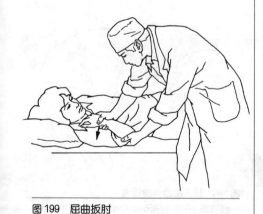

图199 屈曲扳肘
Fig. 199 Flexion-wrenching of the elbow

The manipulation can tense the posterior wall of the elbow capsule, break down the hematoma of the elbow capsule and lead the blood to flow into the interval of the triceps, so as to benefit absorption of the blood. It is adapted to the treatments of the elbow capsule hematoma and the flexion obstruction of the elbow.

2. 桡骨头半脱位复位法

令家长抱住患儿。操作者以一手掌托患肘后部，拇指放于桡骨头上部，其余四指置肘内侧，另一手握患儿前臂下端，两手作对抗拔伸，并逐渐将患儿前臂旋后运动，然后两手配合，一面急速屈曲患肘，一面一手拇指向前顶推桡骨头，即可听到弹响声，示已复位(图200，201)。若上法未能成功，操作者可在轻度牵引下将前臂旋后，另一手拇指则同时向前顶推桡骨小头，两手协调，将肘关节伸直，并将前臂向近端挤压，即可听到弹响声，已示复位(图202)。

2. Reduction of the radius head subluxation

The parent is asked to embrace the suffered child. The physician puts one hand to support the posterior part of the suffered elbow, the thumb on the upper part of the radial head, and the rest fingers on the medial side of the elbow. And holds the lower forearm with other hand to pull and rotate it posterior step by step. Then with the two hands moving coordinately, flexes the elbow rapidly. Meanwhile pushes the radius head directed anteriorly with the thumb. During the manipulation, a spring sound that indicates the joint has been restored can be heard (Fig.200, 201). If the manipulation doesn't get success, the physician can rotate the forearm posteriorly under slight traction, and pushes the radial head directed anteriorly with the thumb at the same time. Then the two hands make a coordinated motion to extend the elbow joint and thrust the forearm directed proximally. If the manipulation is successful, a spring sound can be heard (Fig.202).

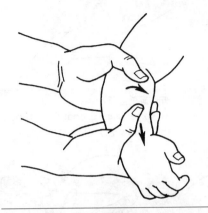

图200 桡骨头半脱位复位法(1)
Fig. 200 Reduction of the radius head subluxation(1)

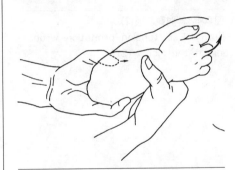

图201 桡骨头半脱位复位法(2)
Fig. 201 Reduction of the radius head subluxation(2)

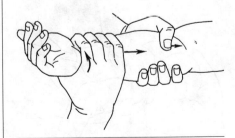

图202 桡骨头半脱位复位法(3)
Fig. 202 Reduction of the radius head subluxation (3)

3. 伸肘旋前扳

操作者以一手掌托肘后部，拇指按压于肘桡侧压痛点，余四指侧置于肘尺侧，另一手握住前臂下端，然后作一快速的大幅度扳动，托肘之手前推，推臂之手后扳并使前臂旋前，将肘

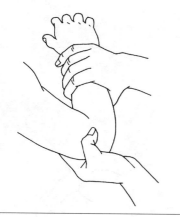

图203 伸肘旋前扳(1)
Fig. 203 Extension-pronation-wrenching of the elbow (1)

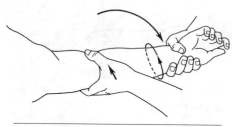

图204 伸肘旋前扳(2)
Fig. 204 Extension-pronation-wrenching of the elbow (2)

关节过伸(图203,204)。本法能牵伸桡侧伸腕肌,分离粘连,适用于肱骨外上髁炎的治疗。

3. Extension-pronation-wrenching of the elbow

The physician puts one palm on the posterior part of elbow to support it, the thumb on the trigger point of radial side and the rest fingers on the ulnar side, and holds the lower part of the forearm with the other hand. Then makes a rapid and broad ranged wrenching, in which the hand that supports the elbow thrusts forward and the hand that holds the forearm wrenches backward and rotates forearm anteriorly to surpass their elastic barrier position a little (Fig.203, 204). This manipulation can tend radial muscles of wrist extension and separate adhesion. It is adapted to the treatment of the tennis elbow.

四、扳胸
Wrenching of the Thoracic Vertebrae

1. 按背扳肩法

患者俯卧。操作者站于胸椎棘突偏凸侧,以靠近患者头端之手掌后豌豆骨抵住偏凸之棘突,另一手抓住对侧肩部向后扳,使胸椎后伸扭转至极限位;然后两手协调用力,作一突发有控制的扳动,扩大扭转幅度3°~5°,并向患者前上方推压棘突,即可听到复位声。本法适用于胸8以上节段胸椎后关节错位及肋椎关节错位的复位(图205)。

1. Wrenching the shoulder while pressing on the dorsum

The patient is in the prone position. The physician stands on the side where the spinous process of the suffered segment is projected. Contacts the spinous process with the pisiform of the wrist which is near the suffered side of the patient, grasps the opposite shoulder to pull it backward, so that the thoracic spine is extended and twisted to its limited position. Then the two hands move coordinately to expand the twisting range in 3 to 5 degree, with one hand wrenching the shoulder and the other thrusting the spinous process. A restoration sound can be heard. This manipulation is adapted to restore those facet joint subluxation, which are above the T8, as

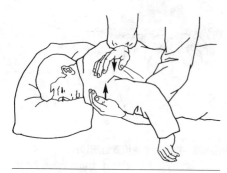

图205 按背扳肩法
Fig. 205 Wrenching the shoulder while pressing on the dorsum

well as the subluxation of costovertebral joints (Fig.205).

2. 按背扳骨盆法

患者体位同上法。操作者以靠近患者头端之手掌后豌豆骨抵住偏凸之棘突，另一手抓住对侧髂前上棘部位向后扳，使脊柱后伸扭转至极限位；然后两手协调用力，作一突发的扳动，扩大扭转幅度3°～5°，并向患者前上方推压棘突，即可复位。本法适用于胸6以下节段的胸椎后关节及肋椎关节错位(图206)。

2. Wrenching the pelvis while pressing on the dorsum

The patient is asked to keep in the same posture as above. The physician contacts the projected spinous process of the suffered segment with the pisiform that is near the rostral side of the patient, grasps the opposite anterior superior iliac spine to pull it backward. Thus the spine is extended and twisted to its limited position. Then the two hands move coordinately to expand twisting range in 3 to 5 degree, with one hand making a sudden wrenching and the other thrusting the spinous process at the superior anterior direction to the patient. The segment can be restored. This manipulation is adapted to those subluxation of the facet joints and the costovertebral joints, which are below the T6 (Fig.206).

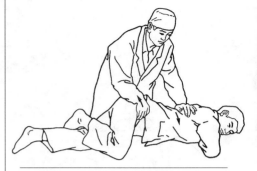

图206 按背扳骨盆法
Fig. 206 Wrenching the pelvis while pressing on the dorsum

3. 旋转定位扳

患者以骑马式跨坐于治疗床上，健侧手靠于胸前，操作者站于其侧后方，一手以拇指顶推偏凸之棘突，另一手从患侧腋下穿过，再以前臂按压其颈后，手推压其对侧肩部，使患者弯腰至病变节段棘间隙张开，再扭转脊柱至弹性限制位，作一突发有控制扳动，扩大扭转幅度3°～5°，同时拇指用力向斜上方顶推棘突，使之复位(图207)。本法适用于胸8以下节段椎骨错缝的整复。

3. Rotation-wrenching of the thoracic vertebrae on selected site

The patient sits on the clinical bed with astride posture, puts his contralateral hand in front of the chest. The physician stands on the laterior posterior side of the patient, presses on the nape with one hand that passing through the patient's opposite armpit and shoulder, while the thumb of the other hand being contacted at the

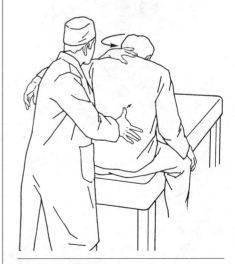

图207 旋转定位扳
Fig. 207 Rotation-wrenching of the thoracic vertebrae on selected site

projected spinous process. Then inducts the patient to flex the waist to the level, at which the interval of spinous processes of the suffered segment is opened, and then the spine rotated to the elastic barrier position. And makes a sudden and controlled wrenching to expand rotation range in 3 to 5 degree, meanwhile the thumb thrusts the spinous process directed medially and superiorly at the same time to get restoration (Fig.207). This manipulation is adapted to the reduction of the thoracic vertebral subluxation, which is below the T8.

4. 双人旋转定位扳

操作方式与上法相似，但两人配合操作。患者坐于凳上。操作者操作方式与上法相同，助手以双腿夹住健侧之大腿，使骨盆固定，两手分置患者两肩前后方，待操作者将脊柱扭转至极限位后，互相配合默契，协助操作者作突发扭转扳动，以求复位（图208，209）。本法适用于体质强健、单人复位无法完成者的手法整复。

4. Rotation-wrenching of the thoracic lumbar vertebrae on selected site by two manipulators

The manipulative manner is similar to above. But it is done by two manipulators. The patient sits on a chair. The physician's action is like above one. The assistant fixes the patient's leg of the healthy side with his two legs, puts two hands on the anterior region of the homolateral shoulder and posterior region of the contralateral shoulder. When the physician rotates the spine to limited position, the assistant helps the physician to make a sudden rotation wrenching, so as to get restoration (Fig.208, 209). This manipulation is suitable for those thoracic vertebral subluxation sufferers whose physiques are too strong to be restored by one manipulator.

5. 侧屈扳法

患者侧卧，胸椎棘突偏凸侧向上。操作者站于其面前，以一手托住颈根部使胸椎侧屈，另一手掌根豌豆骨按压偏凸之棘突并向患者前上方用力，以胸部紧靠患者肩部，使之稳定。当脊柱侧屈至极限后，作一突发有控制的扳动，扩大脊柱侧屈幅度3°～5°，并推压胸椎棘突，使之复位（图210）。本法适用于胸8以上节段椎骨错缝的整复。

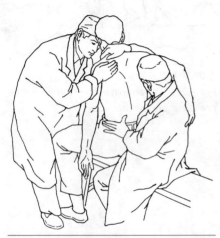

图208 双人旋转定位扳(1)
Fig. 208 Rotation-wrenching of the thoracic lumbar vertebrae on selected site by two manipulators(1)

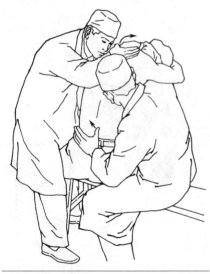

图209 双人旋转定位扳(2)
Fig. 209 Rotation-wrenching of the thoracic lumbar vertebrae on selected site by two manipulators(2)

5. Lateral flexion-wrenching of the thoracic vertebra

The patient is in side lying position, with the projected spinous process of thoracic vertebrae upward. The physician stands in front of the patient, supports the neck bottom with one hand, contacts the projected spinous process and delivers force at the antero-superior direction of the patient with the pisiform of the other hand. Then takes the patient's shoulder to lean against the chest and bend the thoracic spine laterally step by step. When the spine is lateriorly bent to its limited position, makes a sudden and controlled wrenching to expand the range of laterior bending in 3 to 5 degree. At the same time, thrusts the spinous process to get restoration(Fig.210). This manipulation is adapted to the reduction of thoracic vertebral subluxation that is above the T8.

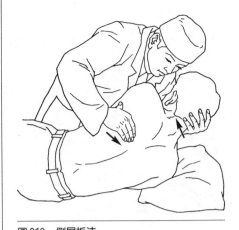

图210 侧屈扳法

Fig. 210 Lateral flexion-wrenching of the thoracic vertebra

6. 坐位推扳法

患者以骑马势坐于治疗床上，两腿分置两侧床缘处，使骨盆固定，双手在胸前交叉抱紧。操作者站于其健侧，一手经胸前抓住患者对侧肩部，使脊柱向健侧扭转并略向上牵引，以松弛肋椎关节；另一手掌根豌豆骨抵住错位肋骨角，作一突发有控制的扳动，扩大旋转幅度3°～5°，同时掌根向患者前外上方推压，使肋骨复位(图211)。本法适用于第8肋以上肋椎关节的整复。

6. Thrusting-wrenching of the thoracic vertebra in sitting position

The patient sits on a clinical bed in astride posture, with his two legs separated on two sides of the bed to fix the pelvis and the arms crossed in front of the chest to hold the opposite shoulders. Standing on the healthy side, the physician grasps the patient's contralateral shoulder with one hand which passes in front of the chest and contacts against the suffered costal angle with the pisiform of the other hand. Then rotates the spine directed healthy side and pulls the spine upward slightly to loosen the costovertebral joints. As the elastic barrier position is attained, makes a sudden and controlled wrenching to expand rotation range in 3 to 5 degree, meanwhile the pisiform thrusting at the anterior laterior superior direction to the patient to cause restoration(Fig.211). This

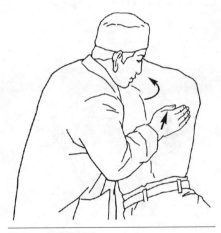

图211 坐位推扳法

Fig. 211 Thrusting-wrenching of the thoracic vertebra in sitting position

manipulation is adapted to the reduction of costovertebral joint that is above T8.

五、扳腰
Wrenching of the Lumbar Vertebrae

1. 斜扳法

斜扳法是目前临床上最常用的一种腰部扳法，并发展了多种变法。最常用的操作方式是令患者侧卧，患侧在上。医生站于其面前，调整肩部与臀部的位置，使脊柱的扭转中心正好落于病变腰椎节段；然后以一手按住肩部向前推，另一上肢肘部半屈，以肘尖和前臂抵住臀部向后扳，将脊柱扭转至弹性限制位后，适时作一突发有控制扳动，扩大扭转幅度3°～5°。可闻到弹响声，示关节面发生相对错移，一般是复位成功的标志(图212)。斜扳法的着力位置也可改在患者屈曲的膝部，以增加扭矩而省力(图213)；或一手穿过屈曲膝关节后侧而扳住下侧大腿(图214)。斜扳法还可在患者背后操作，但改为以肘部向后扳骨盆，以手向前推肩部(图215)。斜扳法适用于腰椎后关节紊乱、急性腰扭伤、腰椎间盘突出症等病症的治疗。

1. Oblique wrenching of the lumbar vertebrae

The oblique wrenching is the most frequently used wrenching of lumbar in clinic. A lot of various manipulative manners have been developed on the basis of the oblique wrenching. The most common manipulative manner is the following one. The patient is in side lying position with the suffered side upward. The physician stands in front of the patient, adjusts the patient's shoulder and buttock location to a suitable position, at which the rotation center of the spine is just on the suffered segment. Then puts one hand on the patient's shoulder and the other flexed elbow and forearm on the buttock. After that, pushes the shoulder forward while wrenchs the buttock backward. When the spine is rotated to its elastic barrier position, makes a sudden and controlled thrusting-wrenching to expand rotation range in 3 to 5 degree. A spring sound that indicates the articular facet is shifted relatively can be heard. Commonly, this is the successful sign of restoration (Fig.212). The contact site may also be changed to the patient's flexed knee so as to

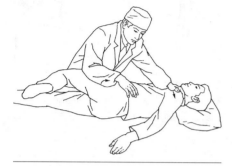

图212 斜扳法(1)
Fig. 212 Oblique wrenching of the lumbar vertebrae (1)

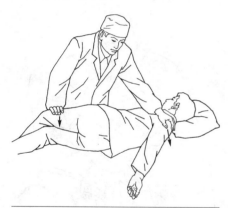

图213 斜扳法(2)
Fig. 213 Oblique wrenching of the lumbar vertebrae(2)

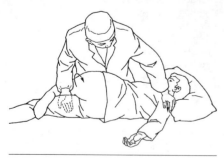

图214 斜扳法(3)
Fig. 214 Oblique wrenching of the lumbar vertebrae(3)

increase twisting distance and laborsaving (Fig.213). Or to the lower side thigh with the hand, which is inserted through the flexed knee (Fig.214). Manipulating behind the patient is also allowed, but the manner is changed into wrenching the pelvis backward and thrusting the shoulder forward (Fig.215). The oblique wrenching is adapted to the treatments of the posterior articulator disturbance of the lumbar vertebrae, the acute sprain of the waist and the protrusion of the lumbar intervertebral disc.

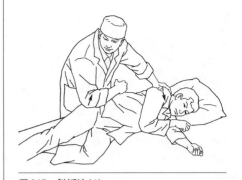

图215 斜扳法(4)
Fig. 215 oblique wrenching of the lumbar vertebrae(4)

2. 改良斜扳法

斜扳法的应用较为盲目，操作者常不能精确估计和控制脊柱的扭转中心，改良斜扳法就是针对这一问题而提出的。患者侧卧，患侧向上。操作者站于其面前，以一手示、中指分触错位节段与上一节段的棘突间隙，另一手抓住患者下侧肩部向前移动，使脊柱轻度屈曲。当手指触及错位节段上一棘突间隙发生扭动，而错位节段下一棘突间尚无相对移动时，停止肩部移动，保持上身体位相对稳定。然后令患者双臂在胸前交叉，抱住对侧肩部。操作者用一手稳定患者肩部，另一手示、中指触摸错位节段和下一节段的棘突间隙，令患者下侧下肢轻度屈髋，使腰椎生理前凸转变为略后突，扩大后关节间隙；屈髋的幅度以触及错位节段下一棘突间隙扩大而错位节段上一棘突间隙保持不动为度。再令患者上侧下肢屈膝屈髋，踝部搁置于下侧下肢膝部，操作者触摸棘突间隙手指改为用指端顶推偏凸棘突，肘部则扳压患者臀部向患侧扭转至极限。此时，脊柱的扭转中心恰好落于错位节段水平，脊柱上下两端杠杆(肩部与骨盆)上进一步增加的扭力，均可导致应力平衡破坏而产生复位移动。操作者适时作一突发有控制的扳动，同时推扳肩部、臀部，并用手指向下推压棘突，即可复位(图216)。斜扳法操作时，推扳动作与患者呼吸配合是有利的。可令患者深呼吸，乘呼气末身体松弛时，作突发扳动。若患者肌肉发达，推扳力量不足以使其复位时，以下方法可增加扭矩，提高复位成功率。①准备动作完成之后，操作者将推肩部之手从患者上侧上肢的腋下穿过，以肘部抵住肩前方前推，示、中指协助另一手的示、中指顶推偏凸之棘突(图217)。②患者侧卧及脊柱扭转的方向与以上手法相反，即向患侧侧卧，而操作者两手手指改为从下而上钩顶偏凸的棘突(图218)。有时患者因向患侧旋转而引起疼痛剧烈而操作困难时，可考虑向健侧旋转复位而用本法。改良斜扳法适用于全腰段椎骨错缝的整复及腰椎间盘突出症的治疗。

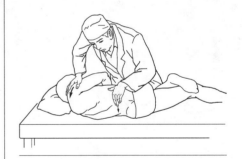

图216 改良斜扳法
Fig. 216 Modified oblique wrenching of lumbar vertebrae

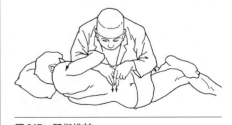

图217 双指推棘
Fig. 217 Thrusting spinous process with two fingers

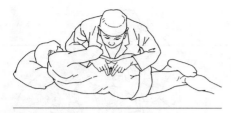

图218 双指勾顶
Fig. 218 Hooking spinous process with two index fingers

2. Modified oblique wrenching of lumbar vertebrae

The manipulative manner of the oblique wrenching is relative sightless. In this wrenching, the manipulator is often unable to estimate control the twisting center of the spine accuracy. Therefore, the modified oblique wrenching is just aimed at this question. The patient is in the side lying position with the suffered side upward. The physician stands in front of the patient, puts the index and middle fingers at the interval of spinous processes that is above the suffered vertebrae and the other below the suffered spinous processes. Then grasps the lower shoulder to move forward and the spine is flexed step by step. If the fingers feel the upper spinous processes moving while lower spinous process keeping in motionless, the physician should stop moving the shoulder and keep the upper trunk in this posture. After that, guides the patient to cross his arms and grasp the opposite shoulders. Fixing up the upper shoulder with one hand, the physician touches the interval of the suffered segment with the index and the middle fingers, and guides the patient to flex the hip joint of the lower side and the lumbar vertebrae so as to expand the intervals of facet joints as well as spinous processes little by little. If the lower interval is expanded while the upper interval is still kept in motionless, the physician should stop flexing the hip and put the patient's ankle of the lower side on the knee of the upper side. With the index finger contacting against the projected process, pushes the patient's shoulder forward with one hand and pull the buttock backward with another elbow to rotate the spine little by little to its limited position. In this way, the twisting center of the spinal column is just located in the suffered segment, and the increased twisting force delivered on both the upper and the lower lever of the spine (the shoulder and the pelvis) may break the stress balance of the spine and give rise to restoration. The physician makes a sudden and controlled wrenching at the suitable time to expand the rotation range in 3 to 5 degree. Meanwhile thrusts the spinous process down with the finger. Thus the subluxation may be corrected (Fig.216). When the modified oblique wrenching is being manipulated, it is benefited to coordinate the wrenching action with breath rhythm of the patient. It is allowed to guide the patient to take deep breath. As the patient's body is loosened at the end of exhalation period, a sudden wrenching is made. If the patient's muscle are very strong and the manipulator's physique is not strong enough to restore the subluxation, one can use the following methods to increase twisting distance and enhance the success rate of restoration. The first one, having the preparative step been accomplished, the physician inserts the hand, which pushes the shoulder in the above manipulative manner, through the armpit to help the fingers of the other hand to thrust the spinous process down with the index and middle fingers, while the elbow pushing the shoulder forward (Fig.217). The second, the direction of side lying and spine rotation is on the contrary of the above manipulative manner, but the other manipulative manner is similar to the above one. The patient's position is changed to lie on suffered side and the physician contact fingers are also changed to hook the projected spinous process low to upward (Fig. 218). If the patient feels severe pain due to homolateral rotation and is unable to be restored, the physician may consider rotating the spine at the contralateral direction to get restoration. The modified oblique wrenching is suitable for the reduction of all articular disturbances of the lumbar vertebrae and the treatment of the protrusion of the lumbar intervertebral disc.

3. 旋转定位扳法

患者以骑马式坐于治疗床上，两腿跨于床缘，使骨盆有效固定；两手手指相扣后抱住枕部，使脊柱上端杠杆组成一体。操作者站于其患侧后方，一手拇指抵住偏凸之棘突，另一手从患侧腋下穿过，经胸前抱住对侧肩部，使患者弯腰扭转；弯腰的幅度视错位的节段而定，腰1错位一般不弯腰，腰2、3错位则略弯腰，腰4、5错位要求弯腰幅度大些。当脊柱扭转至极限位后，适时作一突发扳动，扩大扭转幅度3°～5°，即可复位(图219)。本法适用于腰椎错缝、腰椎间盘突出症的治疗。

3. Rotation-wrenching of lumbar vertebrae on selected site

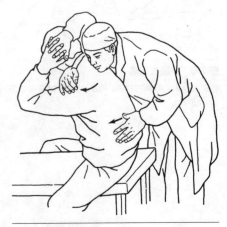

图219 旋转定位扳

Fig. 219 Rotation wrenching of lumbar vertebrae on selected site

The patient rides on a clinical bed with two legs on each side of the bed to fix his pelvis effectively, holds his occiput with crossed fingers of two hands to make the upper lever of the spine as a whole unit. Standing behind the patient, the physician contacts against the projected spinous process with one thumb, grasps the opposite shoulder with the other hand, which inserts through the armpit of suffered side and passes in front of the chest. Then inducts the patient to flex and rotate the spine homolaterally. The flexion range is based on the level of subluxation segment. For the first lumbar vertebra, it isn't required to bend the lumbar. While the L2 and L3, it is required to bend slightly, and the L4 and the L5 to bend at a bigger degree. When the spine is being rotated to its limited position, a sudden wrenching is done to expand the range of rotation at the suitable time, the subluxation can be restored (Fig. 219). This manipulation is adapted to the treatment of the subluxation of the lumbar vertebrae and the protrusion of the lumbar intervertebral disc.

4. 按腰扳腿法

患者俯卧。操作者站于腰椎棘突偏凸侧，一手掌根豌豆骨按抵偏凸之棘突，另一手托住对侧大腿下端向上扳到弹性限制位，然后适时作一突发有控制的扳动，扩大脊柱后伸幅度3°～5°，同时推压棘突，即可复位（图220）。本法适用于腰4、5椎骨错缝及腰椎间盘突出症的治疗。

4. Wrenching leg while pressing on lumbar

The patient is in the prone position. Standing on the suffered side, the physician contacts against the projected spinous process with one pisiform, supports the opposite thigh to pull backward to the spring barrier position with the other hand. Then makes a sudden and controlled wrenching to expand the extension range of the spine in 3 to 5 degree, and thrusting spinous process at the same time. The restoration is gotten (Fig. 220). This manipulation is adapted to the treatments of the vertebral subluxation of L4 and L5, as well as the protrusion of the lumbar intervertebral disc.

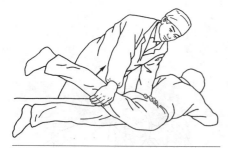

图 220 按腰扳腿法
Fig. 220 Wrenching leg while pressing on lumbar

5. 后伸扳腰法

患者俯卧。操作者脱去鞋子，蹲跨于患者腰部，臀部轻轻触及腰部，以限制脊柱运动；两手抱住患者两大腿向上扳至极限位，作一突发有控制扳动，扩大后伸幅度3°～5°，随即放松，重复操作3～5次(图221)。本法也可改为一膝跪抵腰部，双手握住踝部扳动(图222)。后伸扳腰法适用于腰椎间盘突出症的治疗。

5. Wrenching of lumbar vertebrae by extending lower extremity

The patient is in the prone position. The physician takes off his shoes and squats on the patient's waist to restrict the spine motion with the buttocks contacting against the waist gently. The two hands hold the two thighs of the patient to pull upward to the limited position and make a sudden and controlled wrenching backward to expand the extensive range in 3 to 5 degree. Loosen it at once and repeat the action for 3 to 5 times (Fig.221). This manipulation may also be changed into that manner, in which the physician kneels on the patient's waist with one knee and holds ankle to pull backward with two hands(Fig.222). Extending-wrenching of the lumbar spine is adapted to the treatment of the protrusion of the lumbar intervertebral disc.

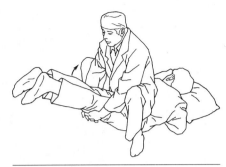

图221 后伸扳腰法(1)
Fig. 221 Wrenching of lumbar vertebrae by extending lower extremity (1)

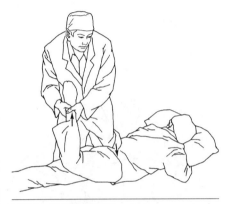

图222 后伸扳腰法(2)
Fig. 222 Wrenching of lumbar vertebrae by extending lower extremity (2)

[附] 滚法与后伸扳腰配合操作
[Appendix] Manipulation of Rolling Coordinated with Wrenching of Lumbar Vertebrae by Extending Lower Extremity.

操作者先以滚法在腰臀两侧予以充分刺激，以缓解疼痛，放松腰部肌肉；然后操作者一手继续在腰部进行滚法操作，另一手托起一侧大腿下端，边滚边后伸大腿至弹性限制位，并作一突发有控制扳动，扩大大腿后伸幅度3°～5°，随即放松(图223)，重复以上动作3～5次；另一侧腰部亦如此操作。本法广泛适用于各种腰腿痛的治疗。

The physician exerts the rolling to stimulate both sides of the waist and buttock fully so as to relieve pain and relax the lumbar muscles. Then, the physician continues carrying on the rolling manipulation on the waist

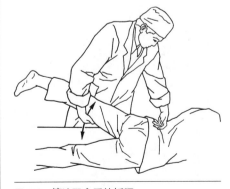

图223 滚法配合后伸扳腰
Fig. 223 Rolling coordinated with wrenching of lumbar vertebrae by extending lower extremity

region with one hand, and supports the lower end of the thigh with the other hand.Extends the thigh step by step to the elastic barrier position and makes sudden and controlled wrenching to expand the extension range of the lumbar in 3 to 5 degree, while rolling.Loosens the thigh immediately(Fig.223) and repeats the above actions for 3 to 5 times.The opposite of the waist is manipulated in the same way. This manipulation is widely used to treat all lumbago and leg pains.

六、扳骶髂关节
Wrenching of Sacroiliac Joint

1. 骶髂关节斜扳法

患者侧卧，患侧向上，下侧下肢伸直，略屈髋，上侧下肢屈膝屈髋。操作者以一手推肩部，使之靠于治疗床；另一手按患者膝部外侧向后下方用力；当脊柱扭转至弹性限制位后，作一突发扳动，将患者膝部向后下方扳压，似扩大骶髂关节间隙，使之在周围韧带弹性力和腘绳肌张力作用下，自行复位。本法适用于骶髂关节向前半脱位(髂后上棘上移、低陷者)的复位(图224)。

1. Oblique wrenching of sacroiliac joint

The patient lies in the side position with the suffered side upward, stretches the knee joint and slightly flexes the hip joint of lower side, flexes the knee and hip joint of the upper side.The physician contacts against the shoulder of upper side to keep it touching on the clinical bed with one hand,and the knee of upper side with the other hand.Then wrenches the knee directed postero-inferiorly to rotate the spine and the sacroiliac joint to its elastic barrier position. Then makes a sudden wrenching, in which the patient's knee is moved adductively and rostrally, so that the interval of the sacroiliac joint is expanded and its facets are shifted by the affects of the spring force of the periarticular ligaments and the tension of the hamstring muscles.This manipulation is adapted to the reduction of anterior subluxation of the sacroiliac joint (the posterior superior iliac spine moves upward and sinks down)(Fig.224).

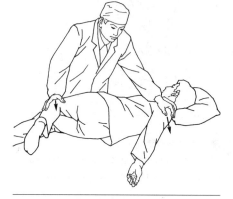

图224 骶髂关节斜扳法
Fig. 224 Oblique wrenching of sacroiliac joint

2. 改良斜扳法

患者体位同上,上侧之手抓住床沿。操作者握住患者下侧手臂向斜上方牵拉,以防止腰椎过度扭曲(图225)。然后令患者松手,两手相抱,抓住对侧肩部,下侧下肢略屈髋,使腰椎生理弧度变为平直;上侧下肢屈膝屈髋,足跟搁置于下侧下肢膝部,骨盆与床面垂直。操作者以一手按患者肩部前推,另一手掌根豌豆骨按于髂后上棘后扳,令患者深吸气后徐徐呼出,在呼气过程中将脊柱扭转。一般经2~3次呼气过程后,即可将脊柱扭转至弹性限制位。在下一次呼气过程中,按肩部之手稳住躯干上部不动,按髂后上棘之手作一突发的扳动,用力方向指向患肢股骨纵轴,即可复位(图226)。本法适用于骶髂关节向后半脱位(髂后上棘下移,后凸)的整复。若整复骶髂关节向前半脱位(髂后上棘上移,低陷),则患者患肢应伸膝屈髋,以利用腘绳肌的杠杆力来帮助复位;扳压部位改为坐骨结节处,用力方向指向患者下颌与下侧肩关节连线的中点;在扳动过程中,操作者可以用自己的大腿移动患者屈髋之大腿,以紧张腘绳肌(图227),增加复位动力。

2. Modified oblique wrenching of sacroiliac joint

The patient is in the same position as above. But grasps the bed edge with the hand of the upper side. The physician holds the arm of lower side to pull directed obliquely superiorly to avoid the lumbar vertebrae being over twisted (Fig. 225). Then the patient is asked to grasps the opposite shoulders with his two arms, flex hip joint of the lower side slightly to make the physiological curvature of the lumbar vertebrae become flat, and keep the pelvis in vertical to the bed surface. With the knee and hip joint of the upper side flexed, the heel of upper side is put on the knee region of the lower side. Later, the physician pushes the upper shoulder to turn forward with one hand, pulls the posterior superior iliac spine to turn backward with the pisiform of the other wrist. Then guides the patient to exhale slowly after deep inhalation and rotate the spine during exhilarative period. Commonly, after 2 to 3 exhalation periods, the spine can be rotated to elastic barrier position. During next exhilarative period, the hand which contacts against the shoulder keep the upper trunk in steady, meanwhile the hand which contacts against the posterior superior

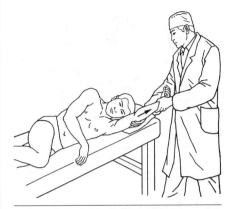

图225 改良斜扳法预备姿势
Fig. 225 Preparatory measures for modified oblique wrenching of sacroiliac joint

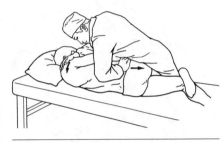

图226 改良斜扳法(1)
Fig. 226 Modified oblique wrenching of sacroiliac joint (1)

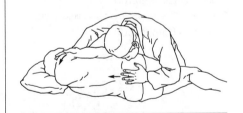

图227 改良斜扳法(2)
Fig. 227 Modified oblique wrenching of sacroiliac joint (2)

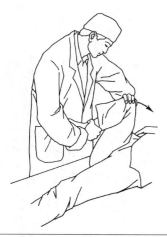

图 228 直腿抬高扳法(1)
Fig. 228 Wrenching of sacroiliac joint by straight lifting leg (1)

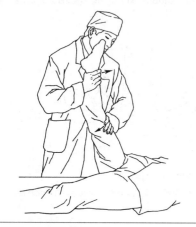

图 229 直腿抬高扳法(2)
Fig. 229 Wrenching of sacroiliac joint by straight lifting leg (2)

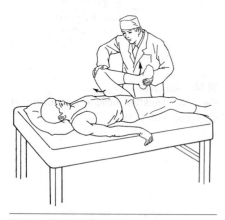

图 230 直腿抬高扳法(3)
Fig. 230 Wrenching of sacroiliac joint by straight lifting leg (3)

iliac spine makes a sudden wrenching directed in the long axis of the femur. Thus the subluxation can be restored (Fig.226). This manipulation is adapted to the reduction of the posterior subluxation of the sacroiliac joint (the posterior superior iliac spine moved downward and bulged posteriorly). For the anterior subluxation (the posterior superior iliac spine moved upward and sinked down), the patient should extend the knee joint and flex the hip joint to take advantage of the lever force of the hamstring muscles to restore the joint, and the contacted point should be changed onto the ischia tuberosity. Then thrusts directed at the middle point of the line between the patient's shoulder of the lower side and the chin. During the thrust course, the physician may move the patient's thigh with one's leg to tend the hamstring muscles and increase reduction impetus(Fig.227).

3. 直腿抬高扳法

患者仰卧。操作者一手握住患肢足跟，另一手按住膝部，将患肢屈膝屈髋，大腿尽量靠近胸腹部(图228)；然后嘱患者咳嗽，待患者咳出，肌肉松弛时，迅速在屈髋状态下将膝关节伸直(图229)。本法适用于腰椎间盘突出症的治疗，亦可整复骶髂关节半脱位。整复骶髂关节半脱位时，若根据半脱位方向而调整髋关节旋转角度则成功率更高。骶髂关节向前半脱位者，屈膝屈髋时将髋关节外旋(膝部旋向外侧，足部旋向内侧，图230)，然后迅速伸直膝关节；骶髂关节向后半脱位者，屈膝屈髋时将髋关节内旋(膝部旋向内侧，足部旋向外侧，图231)，然后迅速伸直膝关节。

3. Wrenching of sacroiliac joint by straight lifting leg

The patient is in the supine position. The physician holds the heel of the suffered side with one hand, presses the knee with the other hand to make the hip and the knee joints flexed and the thigh closed to the chest and the abdomen as possible as it can (Fig.228). Then asks the patient to cough. When the patient coughs out and his muscles are relaxed, rapidly stretches the knee in the flexion condition of hip (Fig.229). This manipulation is adapted to the treatment of the protrusion of the lumbar intervertebral disc, as well as the reduction of the subluxation of the sacroiliac joint. For restoring the subluxation of the sacroiliac joint, if the rotation angle of the hip joint is adjusted on the basis of subluxation type, the success rate will be higher. As restoring the anterior subluxation, the hip joint is lateraly rotated while knee and hip are being flexed (the knee is rotated to lateral side and the foot rotated to medial side, Fig.230). Then the knee joint is rapidly stretched. If the posterior subluxation is restored, the hip joint is medially rotated while the knee and hip joints are being flexed (the knee is rotated medially and the foot rotated lateriorly, Fig. 231). Then the knee joint is rapidly stretched.

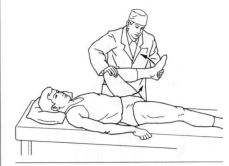

图231 直腿抬高扳法(4)

Fig. 231 Wrenching of sacroiliac joint by straight lifting leg (4)

4. 拽腿扳法

患者仰卧，两手抓住床沿。操作者站于其足端，双手握住患肢踝部，将患肢抬高至45°，并略屈髋屈膝；然后嘱患者咳嗽，待患者咳出，肌肉松弛时，适时作一突发有控制的动作，将患肢向后上方拽拉，使骶髂关节复位(图232)。本法适用于骶髂关节向后半脱位的整复。若患者为向前半脱位，亦可以本法整复，但患肢抬高角度为10°（图233）。

4. Wrenching of sacroiliac joint by pulling flexed lower extremity

The patient lies in supine position and grasps the bed edges with his two hands. The physician stands on the foot side, holds the ankle with hands to lift the suffered leg about 45 degree and make the hip and the knee slightly flexed. Then, asks the patient to cough. As the patient coughs out and his muscles relaxed, makes a sudden and controlled wrenching to draw the leg posterior superiorly. Thus the sacroiliac joint is restored(Fig. 232). This manipulation is adapted to the reduction of the posterior subluxation of the sacroiliac joint. If the patient is anterior subluxation, the manipulation may also be used. But the angle of lifting leg is about 10 degree(Fig.233).

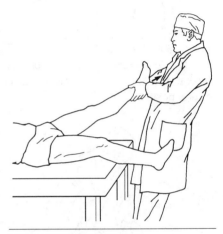

图232 拽腿扳法(后半脱位)

Fig. 232 Wrenching of sacroiliac joint by pulling flexed lower extremity (posterior subluxation)

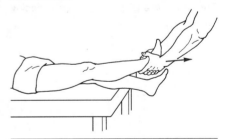

图233 拽腿扳法(前半脱位)

Fig. 233 Wrenching of sacroiliac joint by pulling flexed lower extremity (anterior subluxation)

5. 坐位屈膝屈髋扳法

患儿坐于治疗床端，患肢屈膝屈髋，足踏于床上，健肢自然下垂于床沿。操作者坐于其身后，用双手抱住患儿屈曲之膝部往后上方扳到弹性限制位，作一突发有控制扳动，使骶髂关节复位(图234)。本法适用于小儿骶髂关节错缝的整复。

5. Wrenching of sacroiliac joint by flexing the knee and the hip joints in sitting position

The child sits on the end of clinic bed, flexes the knee and hip joints of suffered side. The homolataral foot is stepped on the bed, whlie the contralateral leg is naturaly hung on bed edge.Sitting behind the child, the physician holds the flexed knee of the child to pull backward and upward to the elastic barrier position with two hands. Then makes a sudden and controlled wrenching to restore the sacroiliac articulatio(Fig.234).This manipulation is adapted to the reduction of child's subluxation of the sacroiliac articulatio.

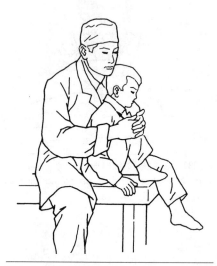

图234 坐位屈膝屈髋扳法
Fig. 234 Wrenching of sacroiliac joint by flexing the knee and the hip joints in sitting position

6. 按骶扳腿法

患者俯卧。操作者站于健侧，一手按住骶骨，另一手托住患肢大腿下端，先使其膝关节屈曲，再将其下肢后伸至弹性限制位，嘱患者咳嗽，趁其咳出，肌肉松弛时，作一突发有控制扳动，扩大下肢后伸幅度3°~5°，即可使骶髂关节复位。本法适用于骶髂关节后脱位的整复(图235)。

6. Wrenching leg while pressing on sacrum

The patient lies in the prone position.Standing on the healthy side, the physician presses the sacrum with one hand and supports the lower part of the suffered thigh with the other hand to makes the knee joint flexed and the leg extended to elastic barrier position at first.Then asks the patient to cough.As the patient is coughing out and the muscles are relaxed, a sudden and controlled wrenching is done to expand the extension range of the leg in 3 to 5 degree.Thus the sacroiliac articulatio can be restored.This manipulation is adapted to the reduction of the posterior subluxation (Fig.235).

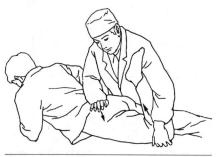

图235 按骶扳腿法
Fig. 235 Wrenching leg while pressing on sacrum

七、扳髋
Wrenching of the Hip

1. 小儿髋关节错缝复位手法

患儿仰卧，操作者站于患侧，以一手按髂前上棘，另一手握大腿下端，将患肢置外展位牵拉，并作轻度摇晃旋转(图236)。有时即可听到复位声响，两下肢恢复等长。若上法复位未成功，操作者可一手握患儿踝部，另一手扶膝部，使之屈髋屈膝，并在髋关节内收位尽量下压，将大腿与腹部相接触。然后作一连续的动作，使髋外展、外旋、伸直下肢，整个动作轨迹如同问号"?"。一般均可在运动过程中听到复位声，同时两下肢恢复等长，说明复位成功。本法适用于小儿髋关节错缝的整复(图237)。

1. Reduction of hip joint subluxation in children

The suffered child lies in the supine position. Standing on the suffered side, the physician presses the anterior superior iliac spine with one hand, holds the lower part of the thigh with the other hand. Then draws the leg in abductive position and slightly waves and rotates it (Fig. 236). Sometimes, a restoration sound can be heard and the two legs may reinstate same length. If the above manipulation doesn't get success, the physician may hold the ankle with one hand and the knee with the other hand to flex the knee and the hip joints, presses the knee under the adductive position as possible as he can to cause the thigh to touch the abdomen. Then makes a series of actions to lead the hip joint to abduct, then to rotate laterally, then to stretch the lower extremity. The locus of the whole course is just like the "?" mark. Generally, a restoration sound can be heard during the motion course, and the two legs may regain same length. It indicates the reduction is successful. This manipulation is adapted to the reduction of the child's subluxation of the hip joint (Fig. 237).

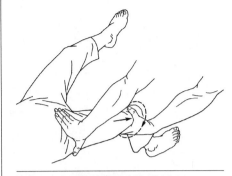

图236 小儿髋关节错缝复位手法(1)
Fig. 236 Reduction of hip joint subluxation in children (1)

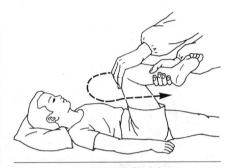

图237 小儿髋关节错缝复位手法(2)
Fig. 237 Reduction of hip joint subluxation in children (2)

2. 成人髋关节错缝复位手法

患者侧卧，患肢屈曲在上，健肢伸直在下。操作者站于其面前，腹部抵住患膝下压，双手环握大腿根部上提片刻，然后将患肢外展、外旋、伸直，术中常可听"咯吱"声，示已复位(图238)。若未获成功，不可反复操作，可隔日再治，本法适用于成人髋关节错缝的复位。

2. Reduction of hip joint subluxation in adults

The patient lies on the healthy side, with the suffered leg flexed and the healthy leg stretched. Standing in front of the patient, the physician holds the upper end of the thigh to lift it for a while, contacts against the knee to press it downward with his abdomen. Then makes the

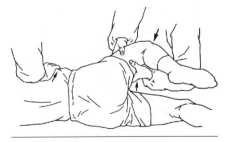

图238 成人髋关节错缝复位手法
Fig. 238 Reduction of hip joint subluxation in adults

suffered leg abducted then laterally rotated and then stretched. During this course, a "gezhi" sound can often be heard. It indicates that the joint is restored (Fig.238). If the manipulation isn't got success, you needn't repeat this manipulation again, but it is allowed to treat in two days latter. This manipulation is adapted to the reduction of the adult's subluxation of the hip joint.

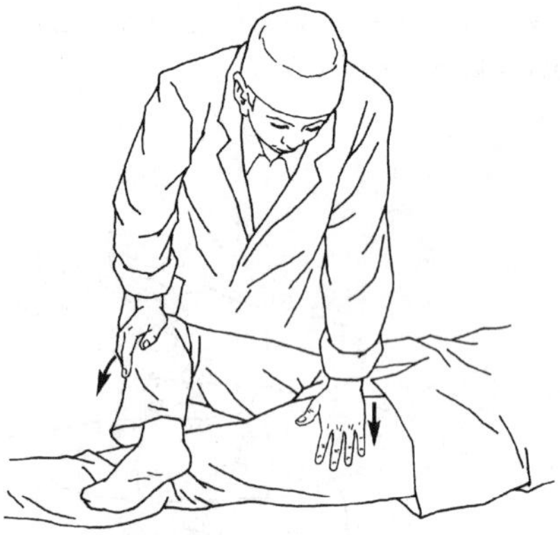

3. "4"字扳法

患者仰卧，患肢屈髋外旋外展屈膝，足跟搁置于健肢膝部，成"4"字形。操作者站于患侧，一手按对侧髂前上棘处，另一手按于患膝下压，逐渐将髋关节外展外旋至弹性限制位；然后作一突发有控制扳动，扩大髋外展外旋幅度3°～5°，随即放松，重复以上操作3～5次。本法适用于内收肌劳损、髋关节滑囊炎的治疗(图239)。

3. Wrenching of hip joint as constrained Patrick's test

Lying in the supine position, The patient flexes, laterally rotates and abducts the hip, flexes the knee of the suffered leg, and puts the heel on the healthy knee to form a "4" mark. Standing on the suffered side, the physician presses the opposite anterior superior iliac spine with one hand, pushes the knee downward with the other hand gradually, so as to make the hip joint abducted and laterally rotated to elastic barrier position. Then makes a sudden and controlled wrenching to expand the abductive and lateriorly rotation range of the hip joint in 3 to 5 degree. Loosens the hip immediately. Repeats the above action for 3 to 5 times. This manipulation is adapted to the treatment of the strain of the adductor muscles and the bursal synovitis of hip (Fig. 239).

图239 "4"字扳法
Fig. 239 Wrenching of hip joint as constrained Patrick's test

[附] 滚法与髋关节扳法配合操作
[Appendix] Manipulation of Rolling Coordinated with Wrenching of Hip

1. 滚法配合髋内旋扳法

患者俯卧，操作者先在臀部充分使用滚法操作，然后一手继续在梨状肌体表部位进行滚法刺激，另一手握患肢踝部，使之屈膝后向外扳至疼痛限制位(髋内旋),并作一突发有控制的扳动,扩大内旋幅度3°～5°,随即放松。重复以上操作3～5次(图240)。本法适用于梨状肌综合征治疗。

1. Rolling coordinated with medial rotation wrenching of hip joint

The patient is in the prone position. The physician delivers rolling on the buttocks over and over at first. Then while imposing rolling stimulus on the piriform's area with one hand, holds the ankle to flex the suffered side and pull the angle directed laterally to painful barrier position (medial rotation of the hip) with the other hand. At this moment, makes a sudden and controlled wrenching to expand medial rotation range in 3 to 5 degree, and loosens immediately. Repeats the above action for 3 to 5 times(Fig.240). It is adapted to the treatment of pisiform syndrom.

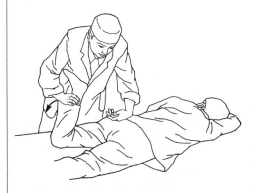

图240 滚法配合髋内旋扳法

Fig. 240 Rolling coordinated with medial rotation wrenching of hip joint

2. 滚法配合"4"字扳

患者仰卧,患肢足跟搁置于健肢膝部成"4"字形。操作者先在其腹股沟部、内收肌部位充分实施滚法操作。然后一手继续在腹股沟部、内收肌部位进行滚法刺激,另一手按患膝下压至疼痛限制位,作一突发有控制的扳动,扩大髋外展外旋幅度3°～5°,随即放松,重复以上操作3～5次(图241)。本法适用于内收肌劳损、髋关节滑囊炎、腰3横突综合征的治疗。

2. Rolling coordinated with wrenching of hip joint as inforced Patrick's test

The patient is in the supine position, puts the heel of the suffered lower limb on the knee of the healthy side to form a "4" mark. The physician exerts the rolling manipulation on the region of groin, adductor muscles at first. Then going on the rolling stimulus on these regions with one hand, pushes the suffered knee downward to painful barrier position with the other hand. At this moment, makes a sudden and controlled thrusting to expand the abduction and lateral rotation range of the hip in 3 to 5 degree, and loosens the hip immediately. Repeats the above manipulation for 3 to 5 times(Fig. 241). This manipulation is adapted to the treatments of the strain of the adductor muscles, the bursitis of the hip joint and the syndrome of the transverse process of the

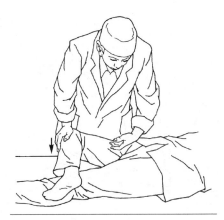

图241 滚法配合"4"字扳

Fig. 241 Rolling coordinated with wrenching of hip joint as inforced Patrick's test

third lumbar vertebrae.

八、扳膝
Wrenching of Knee

1. 屈膝扳法

患者仰卧。操作者一手扶患肢膝部，另一手握踝部，逐渐将膝关节屈曲至疼痛限制位，然后作一突发有控制扳动，扩大屈膝幅度3°~5°。本法适用于髌上囊积液、膝关节周围粘连症的治疗(图242)。

1. Flexion-wrenching of knee

The patient is in the supine position. The physician supports the suffered knee with one hand, holds the ankle with the other hand to force the knee joint to be flexed to painful barrier position gradually. Then makes a sudden and controlled action to expand the range of flexion in 3 to 5 degree. This manipulation is adapted to the treatments of the effusion of the suprapatellar bursa and the adhesion syndrome of the perigenual articulatio (Fig.242).

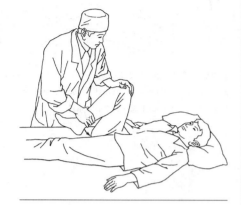

图242 屈膝扳法
Fig. 242 Flexion-wrenching of knee

2. 伸膝扳法

患者体位与操作者姿势同上法，将膝关节伸直至疼痛限制位后两手协调用力，一手下压膝部，一手上提踝部，突发有控制地扩大伸膝幅度3°~5°。本法适用于膝关节周围粘连症的治疗(图243)。

2. Extension-wrenching of knee

The patient's position and the physician's posture both are the same as above. The physician stretches the suffered knee joint to painful barrier position. Then suddenly and controlled expands the extension range of the knee in 3 to 5 degree, with one hand thrusting the knee down and the other hand wrenching the ankle up. This manipulation is adapted to the treatment of the adhesion syndrome of the perigenual articulatio(Fig.243).

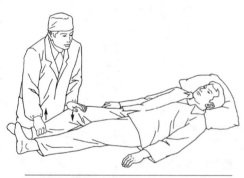

图243 伸膝扳法
Fig. 243 Extension-wrenching of knee

3. 屈膝推扳法

患者俯卧，患膝屈曲成90°，与床沿齐，双手抓住前床沿。操作者俯身于其足端，将其足背搭在肩上，两手握住小腿上端；先沿胫骨纵轴上提、下压数次，再沿股骨纵轴前推、后扳数次，并将小腿左右扳动数次；然后再沿股骨纵轴向远端牵拉的同时，将小腿内旋—屈曲—外旋—伸直，再作外旋—屈曲—内旋—伸直。本法适用于膝关节紊乱症的治疗(图244)。

3. Thrusting-wrenching of knee in flexion position

Lying in the prone position, the patient keeps his suffered knee in 90 degree of flexion and out of the bed edge, and grasps the opposite edge of the bed with his hands. Standing on the foot side with his trunk leaning forward, the physician takes the patient's instep on his shoulder, holds the upper part of lower leg with hands to pull it up at first and then push it down along the long axis of the tibia for several times. Next, pushes the lower leg forward and pull it backward for several times along the long axis of the femur. After then, shakes the lower leg from right to left and from left to right for several times. Finally, inducts the knee joint to be rotate medially, then to be flexed, then to be rotated laterally and last to be stretched while the knee is kept in truction along the long axis of the femur. Repeats the above action conterdirected, i.e. lateral rotation, then flexion, then medial rotation and last extension again. This manipulation is suitable for the treatment of the articular disturbance of the knee (Fig.244).

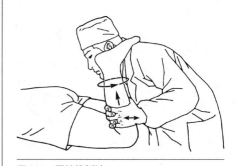

图244　屈膝推扳法

Fig. 244　Thrusting-wrenching of knee in flexion position

[附] 滚法配合膝关节扳法操作
[Appendix] Manipulations of Rolling Coordinated with Wrenching of Knee

患者仰卧。操作者先在股四头肌、膝关节周围施以滚法操作，以缓解局部疼痛与肌肉紧张；然后操作者一手继续在两膝眼处予以滚法刺激，另一手握住踝部，边滚边将膝关节屈曲至疼痛限制位，并作一突发有控制扳动，扩大屈曲幅度3°～5°，然后放松；重复以上操作3～5次(图245)。然后令患者俯卧，膝下垫以软枕，一手在腘窝部施滚法刺激，另一手握住踝部逐渐伸膝至疼痛限制位，再作突发扳膝动作，扩大伸膝幅度3°～5°，随即放松。重复以上操作3～5次(图246)。本法适用于膝关节疼痛、积液、屈伸不利的治疗。

The patient is in the supine position. The physician

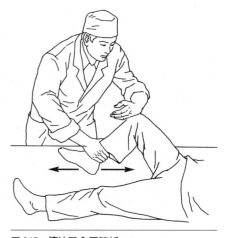

图245　滚法配合屈膝扳

Fig. 245　Rolling coordinated with flexion-wrenching of knee

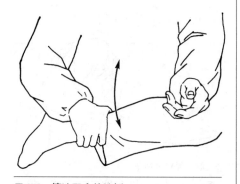

图246 拨法配合伸膝扳
Fig. 246 Rolling coordinated with extension—wrenching of knee

applies rolling manipulation on the quadriceps femoris region and the knee region to relieve local pain and muscle contraction at first. Exerting rolling stimulus on the dimples beneath patella continually with one hand, the physician holds the ankle with the other hand to flex the knee to painful barrier position while rolling. Then thrusts suddenly and controllably to expand flexion range in 3 to 5 degree and loosens the knee immediately. The above motion is repeated for 3 to 5 times (Fig.245). Latter,guides the patient to lie prostrately and put a soft pillow under his knee.While exerting rolling on the hollow of the knee with one hand,the physician holds the ankle with the other hand to extend the knee to painful barrier position gradually. Then makes a sudden and controlled thrust to expand the extensional range of knee in 3 to 5 degree.Loosens immediately and repeats the above action for 3 to 5 times(Fig.246).These manipulations are adapted to the treatment of the knee pain, the effusion of the genuarticular cavity, as well as the inconvenient flexion–extension of the knee.

九、扳足踝
Wrenching of Ankle and Foot

1. 扳踝关节

患者仰卧。操作者站于其足端，一手托住其足跟，另一手握住足趾部，两手协调，先将踝关节逐渐背伸至疼痛限制位，随即作一突发有控制扳动，扩大背伸幅度3°～5°。接着将踝关节按上述操作方式向跖屈、内翻、外翻方向扳动(图247)。本法适用于踝关节扭伤、踝关节骨关节炎等病症的治疗。

1. Wrenching of ankle

The patient is in the supine potion.Standing on the foot side, the physician supports the heel with one hand, holds the forefoot and toes with the other hand.With the two hands coordinately manipulating, then the physician inducts the ankle joint to be extended gradually to painful barrier position. And at this moment, makes a sudden and controlled wrenching to expand the extensional range in 3 to 5 degree. Later, inducts the ankle joint to

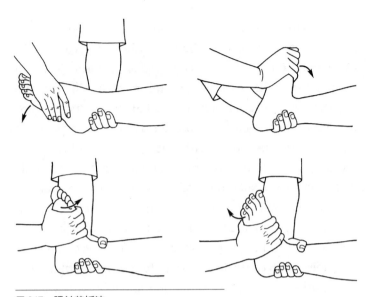

图247 踝关节扳法
Fig. 247 Wrenching of ankle

be flexed, to be supinated, and to be pronated according to the above manipulative manner (Fig 247). This manipulation are adapted to the treatments of the sprain of the ankle joint and the osteoarthritis of the ankle.

2. 距下关节错位复位法

患者坐床上,足踝部超出床沿,并视距下关节错位类型,将内踝(内翻型)或外踝(外翻型)贴紧床面。一助手固定小腿上部,操作者一手由后跟向前握住足跟,另一手由足底向后握住足跟,双手拇指重叠按压距跟关节的外侧(内翻型)或内侧(外翻型),余指重叠托提距跟关节内侧(内翻型)和外侧(外翻型)。先将跟骨沿胫骨纵轴向远端牵拉片刻;再使患足背屈,改为沿跟骨纵轴向远端拔伸并尽量将患足内翻(内翻型)和外翻(外翻型);保持片刻后,突然将患足外翻(内翻型)或内翻(外翻型),拇指用力向近端及下方推压,余指向远端及上方托提,呈一捻动作,使距下关节复位(图248,249)。本法适用于距下关节错缝的整复。

2. Reduction of the subtalar joint subluxation

Sitting on the clinical bed, the patient keeps his ankle and feet stretching out of the bed and the medial malleolus (supination subluxation) or the lateral malleolus (pronation subluxation) putting against the bed surface, on the basis of the subluxation type of the subtalar joint. An assistant fixes the lower leg. The physician holds the heel from

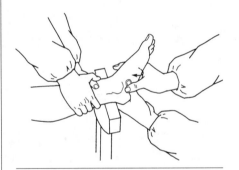

图248 距下关节错位复位法(外翻型)
Fig. 248 Reduction of subtalar joint subluxation (Supinational type)

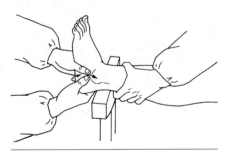

图249 距下关节错位复位法(内翻型)
Fig. 249 Reduction of subtalar joint subluxation (Pronational type)

heel side to toe side with one hand and from sole side to heel side with the other hand, while the two thumbs overlapped on the lateral side of talocalcanean joint (in supination subluxation) or the medial side of the talocalcanean joint (in pronation subluxation) and the rest fingers overlapped on the opposite side to force the subtalar joint to be turned downward. After pulling the heel along the long axis of the tibia for a minute, makes the ankle flexed and then pulls the heel along the long axis of the calcaneum while the foot kept in supination position (supination subluxation) or in pronation position(pronation subluxation) to the greatest range. At this moment, makes a sudden and controled motion to pronate (supination subluxation)or supinate (pronation subluxation) the suffered foot. Meanwhile thrusts the calcaneum directed proximally inferiorly with the thumbs and wrenchs the calcaneum directed distally superiorly with the rest fingers. The whole action is as a screw. Thus the subtalar joint is restored(Fig.248, 249). This manipulation is adapted to the reduction of the subtalar joint subluxation.

3. 距舟关节错位复位法

患者卧位，并根据舟骨移位方向而将足该侧朝上(内移型足内侧朝上，背移型足背侧朝上，跖移型尽量将足心朝上)。一助手固定踝部，另一助手握跖趾部沿足纵轴方向向远端牵拉。操作者以双手拇指重叠按压于舟骨移位侧，余手指托提于对侧；令助手相对牵引患足片刻后，逐渐将患足转变成导致舟骨移位的姿势(如内移型者成外展位，背移型者成跖屈位，跖移型者成背屈位)，至极限位后，三人协调动作，突然将患足姿势向反方向扳动(外展位成内收位，跖屈位成背屈位，背屈位成跖屈位)，术者拇指同时推压舟骨，即可复位(图250，251)。本法适用于距舟关节错位的整复。足部其他小关节错缝亦可仿本法予以复位。

3. Reduction of the talonavicular joint subluxation

Lying on a clinic bed on the basis of the navicular subluxation type, the patient puts the shifting side of the foot upward (the medial side of the foot is put upward for the medial subluxation type, the instep is put upward for dorsal subluxation type, the sole is put upward for plantar subluxation type). One assistant fixes the ankle,

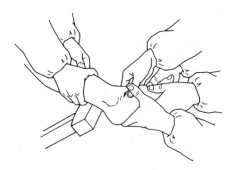

图250 距舟关节复位法(内移型)
Fig. 250 Reduction of talonavicular joint subluxation (medial subluxation type)

another assistant holds the plantar and toe to pull along the long axis of the foot with hands. The physician's thumbs overlapped press at the point, at which the navicular is projected, while the rest fingers on the opposite side. Guides the assistants relatively to pull the foot for a minute, and then gradually to change the foot into that posture in which the talonavicular subluxation was happened, (For example, make the foot of medial subluxation in abduction position, make the foot of the dorsal subluxation in plantar flexion position and make the foot of plantar subluxation in dorsal flexion position). As the elastic barrier position is gotten, the three persons coordinate their actions to wrench the foot at the opposite direction suddenly (abduction into adduction, plantar flexion into dorsal flexion and dorsal flexion into plantar flexion). And the physician's thumb thrust the navicular at this moment. Thus the joint can be restored (Fig. 250, 251). This manipulation is adapted to the reduction of the talonavicular joint subluxation. The subluxation of the rest minor joints of the foot may be restored with a similar manipulation.

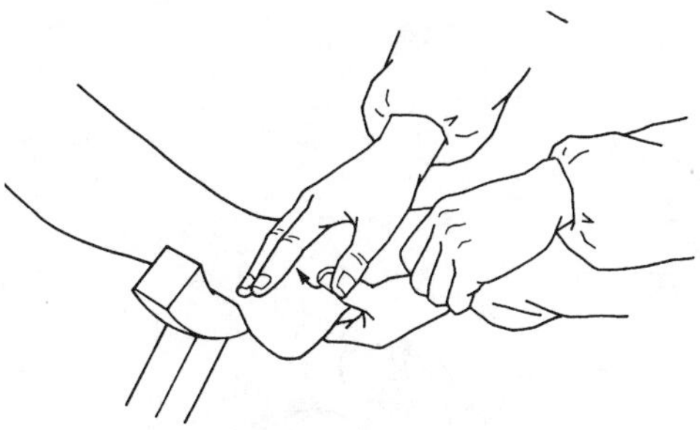

图 251 距舟关节复位法（跖移型）
Fig. 251 Reduction of talonavicular joint subluxation (plantar subluxation type)

第十一节　背顶类手法

SECTION 11 CATEGORY OF COUNTERWORKING MANIPULATIONS

所谓背顶类手法是指以物固定脊柱一点，并利用与该点不在同一水平上的反向剪切力使脊柱后伸，以达到整复关节错位或促进髓核回纳的一类手法操作。背顶类手法可用图252模拟表示。

The so-called "category of counterworking manipulations" means those actions in which the spine is fixed at a point and extended by a sharing force at opposite direction which isn't at the same level of the

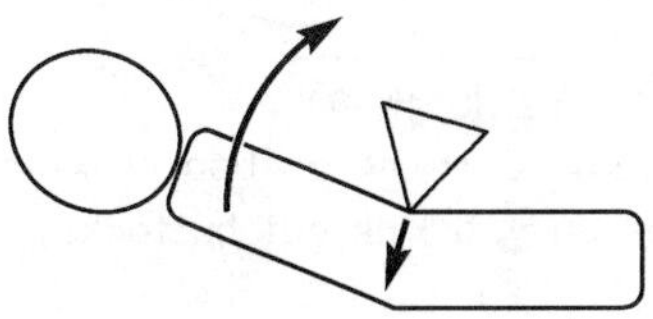

图 252 背顶类手法模式图
Fig. 252 Model of category of counterworking manipulation

point, so as to reset joint subluxation or promote the nuclear of the disc being reverted. These manipulations can be modeled with the Fig.252.

一、背法
Carrying on Back

1. 背法

患者与操作者相背站立，操作者两臂从患者腋下伸入，以屈曲的肘部勾住患者肘部并将其背起。嘱患者肌肉放松，头颈尽量靠近操作者背部。先停顿片刻，使患者因脊柱过伸而产生的腰痛加剧有所缓解，并利用自身重力，牵拉患者脊柱，减轻肌紧张。然后慢慢将患者身体下滑，使患部对准操作者骶尾部，再作小幅度的左右晃抖动作，使患者身体随之抖动(图253)；待患者肌肉松弛时，作一突发的伸膝挺臀动作，使患者脊柱震动，产生关节面移动而复位。本法适用于腰椎后关节紊乱、腰椎间盘突出症的治疗(图254)。

1. Carrying on back

The patient and the physician stand back by back. The physician hooks the patient's elbow with his flexed elbow to lift the patient up. Then asks the patient to relax muscles and lean the head against his back as possible as he can. The patient body is kept in still for a while to relieve the pain caused by the overextension of the spine, so that takes advantage of the weight of the patient body to pull the spine downward and relieve muscle tension first. Then the patient's body is slip down slowly to that condition in which ones suffered part and the physician's sacro coccyx joint are contacted. Later, the physician shakes the buttocks left and right to make the patient's body swing in space (Fig.253). When the patient's muscles are relaxed, the physician makes a sudden motion in which his knee is extended and his buttocks are stuck out to shake the patient's spine, so that the joint facets are shifted and reverted. This manipulation is adapted to treatments of facet joint disorder of the lumbar vertebrae and the protrusion of the lumbar intervertebral discs (Fig. 254).

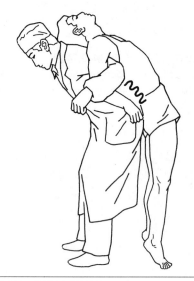

图253 背法(牵拉晃抖)
Fig. 253 Carrying on back (pulling and shaking)

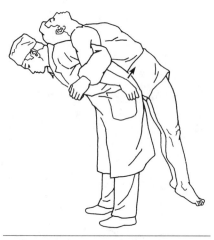

图254 背法(挺臀伸膝)
Fig. 254 Carrying on back (extending knees and sticking out buttocks)

2. 侧背法

背法也可这样操作：操作者以一手从患者健侧腋下伸过，从胸前抱住患者身体，以髂嵴为支点，将患者侧背起（图255）；停顿片刻后，适时作一抖胯动作，使者脊柱震动而产生复位移动。本法适用于腰椎后关节紊乱的整复。

2. Lateral carrying on back

The manipulation, carrying on back can also be manipulated as follows: The physician inserts his arm through the armpit of the healthy side and holds the patient's body. Then takes the iliac-crest as fulcrum to lift the body up(Fig.255). Had the patient's body kept in still for a while, a sudden buttock motion of shaking is done by the physician so as to come into restoration shifting. This manipulation is adapted to rectify the disorder of lumbar facet joint.

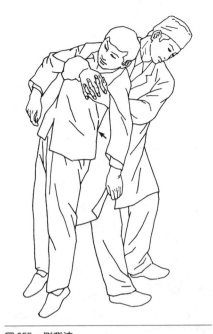

图255 侧背法
Fig. 255 Lateral carrying on back

二、对抗复位法
Antagonistic Reduction of Thoracic Vertebrae

患者坐位，双手十指相扣，抱于枕部。操作者站于其身后，以与患侧同侧之足踏于患者坐椅，膝部抵住胸椎棘突偏凸处下缘，两手从患者屈曲的肘关节内穿入，抓住腕部，将其向后扳拉至限制位，然后嘱其深呼吸；待患者呼气肌肉放松时，适时作一突发有控制的扳动，利用一对方向相反、不在同一平面上的剪切力，使小关节复位。本法适用于胸4至胸10节段胸椎后关节及肋椎关节错位的治疗（图256）。

The patient is in the sitting position, with his fingers of two hands crossed to hold the occiput. Standing behind the patient, the physician contacts against the lower rim of the projected spinous process of the suffered segment with the knee, while the foot of the same side is stepped on the bench. Then inserts his two hands through the patient's flexed elbows and holds the wrist to pull backward to the limit position. Later, asks the patient to take deep breath. If the patient is exhaling and his muscles are relaxing, makes sudden and controlled wrenching and thrusting to restore the facet joint by utilizing a double shearing forces that are in the opposite directions but not at the same level. This manipulation is adapted to the

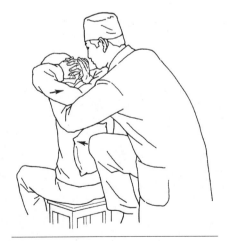

图256 对抗复位法
Fig. 256 Antagonistic reduction of thoracic vertebrae

treatments of the subluxation of the thoracic vertebral facet joint which located from the T4 to the T10, as well as the subluxation of the costoverebral joints (Fig.256).

三、顶法
Counterworking

1. 仰卧位顶法

患者仰卧，背部垫一弹性垫子，使其身体略向前上倾斜，双臂交叉于胸前，手抓住对侧肩部而相抱，使胸廓组成一个整体而更趋稳定。操作者站于患侧，一手握拳垫于错缝之胸椎后关节或肋椎关节的下缘，一手推患者胸前相抱之手臂使脊柱后伸至极限位；随后嘱患者深呼吸，待呼气期肌肉放松时，适时作一突发有控制推压，扩大脊柱后伸幅度3°～5°，即可复位（图257）。此法患者容易放松，较为安全，适合于孕妇、年老、体弱多病者胸椎错缝或肋椎关节错缝的整复。

1. Counterworking in supine position

With a spring cushion put under his back, the patient lies in the supine position, inclined his thunk anterior-superiorly, and crosses his two arms in front of the chest to grasp the opposite shoulders with the hands to make the thoracic frame become a integration and more steady. The physician stands on the suffered side. With his fist put under the lower rim of the suffered facet joint of the thoracic vertebra or costoverebral joint, pushes elbows of the patient's crossed arms forward to extend the spine to its limit position with the other hand. Then asks the patient to take deep breath. During the exhalation period when the muscle is being relaxed, thrusts the elbows suddenly and controllably to expand the extension range of the spine in 3 to 5 degree. Thus the joint is restored (Fig.257). The sufferer is easy relaxed and more safely in this manipulation. Those aged or feeble patients as well as prognant women who are suffered from the subluxation of thoracic facet joint or the costoverebral joint are suitable for this manipulation.

2. 坐位顶法

患者坐位，身体略后仰，其他姿势同上法。操作者坐于其

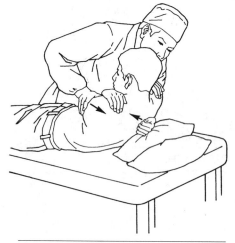

图257 仰卧位顶法
Fig. 257 Counterworking in supine position

身后，在患者后背与操作者胸前置一圆形弹力垫，垫的位置正好位于错缝关节之下缘；操作者用双手抱住患者两肘部向后上方用力扳拉，使脊柱受轻度牵拉并后伸至限制位；嘱患者深呼吸，乘其呼气期肌肉放松时，适时作一突发有控制扳拉，同时胸部前顶，使关节复位(图258)。本法适用于胸8以上节段椎骨错缝和肋椎关节错缝的整复。

2. Counterworking in sitting position

The patient sitts on a bench and extends the trunk slightly. Sitting behind the patient, the physician put a globose cushion between the patient and the physician's bodies. The location of this cushion is just at the lower rim of the suffered joint. Then the physician holds two elbows of the patient to pull them posteriorly and superiorly. In this way, the spine is extended and hauled to its limit position. Later the patient was asked to take deep breath. When the patient is exhaling and his muscles are being relaxed, the physician wrenches the patient trunk backward suddenly and controllably while counterworks against the back with the chest to restore the joint (Fig.258). The manipulation is adapted to the reduction of thoracic facet joint subluxation and costoverebral joint subluxation which are above the level of T8.

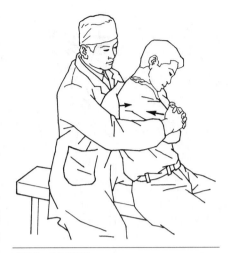

图258 坐位顶法
Fig. 258 Counterworking in sitting position

3. 立位顶法

患者站立，身体后仰，其他姿势同前二法。操作者站于其身后，在患者后背与操作者胸前置一圆形弹性垫，其高度位于错位关节的下缘。然后操作者按坐位顶法的操作方式，扳顶胸椎而使之复位(图259)。本法适用于胸8以上节段椎骨错缝及肋椎关节错缝的整复。

1. Counterworking in standing position

Being standing position, the patient inclines his tunk posteriorly. His other postures are the same as above. Sitting behind the patient, the physician put a globose cushion between the patient and the physician's bodies. The location of this cushion is just at the lower rim of the suffered joint. Then according to the manipulative manner as above, wrenches and sticks against the thoracic vertebra to make restoration (Fig.259). The indications of this manipulation are the same as the above one.

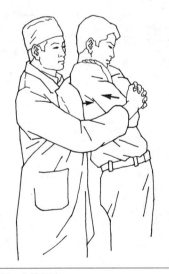

图259 立位顶法
Fig. 259 Counterworking in standing position

四、踩跷法
Stepping

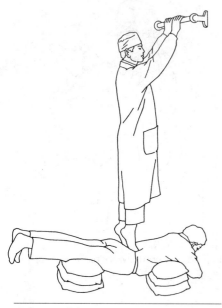

图260 踩跷法
Fig. 260 Stepping

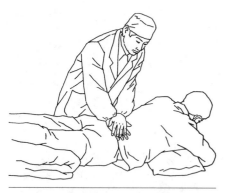

图261 按压振腰法
Fig. 261 Pressing-vibrating of lumbar

患者俯垫，在其胸前及骨盆处各用几个枕头相叠垫起，使脊柱过伸，腹部悬空。操作者双手抓住墙上扶杆，以承受自己的体重；轻轻将两足尖踩踩于患者腰部；然后嘱患者正常呼吸，操作者根据患者呼吸周期而有节律地弹跳，吸气时轻轻跳起，呼气时轻轻落下，但足尖不能离开患者腰部，以免形成冲击力(图260)。根据患者体质强弱，可逐渐加重(目前已少用)弹跳力量，以患者能忍受为限，一般弹跳5～10次即可。本法适用于腰椎间盘突出症的治疗。踩跷法的足尖弹跳运动也可用双手有节律的短促按压动作来代替，这样用力的大小和幅度较容易控制，但该法不再称为踩跷法，而称为按压振腰法(图261)。

The patient is in the prone position, with a few pillows under his chest and pelvis to make his spine be overextended and his abdomen suspended. The physician steps gently on the patient's waist with his toes, while holds a handrail which is fixed on the wall to support his weight. Then asks the patient to take deep breath. If the patient's muscle is relaxed, the physician springs up and drops down according to the respiratory cycles rhythmically. i.e. leaps up gently in the inhalation period and falls down in the exhalation period. Pay attention on that the toes mustn't leave the lumbar in order to avoid shocking force that may cause trauma (Fig.260). It is allowed to increase the springing force gradually on the basis of the patient's constitution, but not beyond the patient's endurance. Commonly, one can repeat springing for 5 to 10 times. This manipulation is adapted to the treatment of the protrusion of the lumbar intervertebral disc. The spring motion of the toes in stepping may be replaced with rhythmic, brief thrusting motion of the hands. In this way, the magnitude of force and range of the spring are controlled easily. But this manipulation is called as the pressing-vibrating of lumbar (Fig.261), not called as the stepping yet, which now is seldom used.

第十二节 拔伸类手法
SECTION 12 CATEGORY OF PULLING-STRETCHING MANIPULATIONS

所谓拔伸类手法是指对患者病变肢体进行纵向牵拉的一类操作。拔是指手法操作时的动作，伸是指手法所产生的伸长效应。拔伸类手法可用图262模拟表式。

The so-called "category of pulling-stretching manipulations" refers to those actions in which the suffered limb (or trunk) is pulled along its long axis. Pulling means the motion of the manipulations, while stretching means the expanding effect of the manipulations. These manipulations can be modeled with Fig.262.

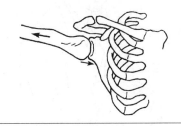

图262 拔伸类手法模式图
Fig. 262 Model of category of pulling-stretching manipulations

一、拔颈项
Pulling of the Neck

1. 虎口托颌拔颈法

患者坐位。操纵者站于其后，两手虎口张开，以拇指和示指虎口缘抵住下颌骨与枕骨下缘抱紧，两前臂尺侧缘置肩上；然后以前臂为杠杆，肩部为支点，肘部下压，双手上托，将颈部向上牵拉（图263）。在拔伸颈项的同时，可配合颈部小幅度屈伸、摇转、侧屈运动。本法适用于颈项僵硬疼痛、屈伸不利的治疗。

1. Pulling of the neck by supporting jaw with thumb web

The patient is in the sitting position. The physician stands behind the patient, supports the patient's jaw and occiput with opened first webs of hands, and puts the ulnar sides of forearms on the patient's shoulders. Then takes the forearm for lever, and the shoulder for fulcrum to draw the head upward, with the elbow pressing down and the hands pulling up(Fig.263). While pulling the neck, one can coordinate with flexion-extension, rotation and lateral bending movements of the neck. This

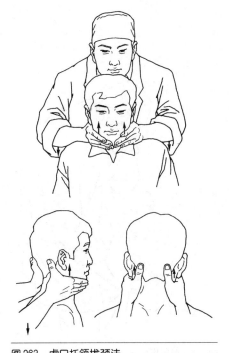

图263 虎口托颌拔颈法
Fig. 263 Pulling of neck by supporting jaw with thumb web

manipulation is adapted to the treatments of stiff neck, inconvenient motion of neck and cervical spondylopathy.

2. 前臂托颌拔颈法

患者坐位。操作者站于其后，以一侧手臂从患者颈前绕过，托起下颌，其手按压于患者对侧肩上；另一手虎口张开，托住患者枕部；然后以托下颌之前臂为杠杆，肩部为支点，将患者头部向上牵拉，另一手则保持头颈处于中立位(图264)。在牵拉过程中，托下颌之前臂可作突发有控制的小幅度左右晃抖动作，使颈椎左右旋转。本法适用于颈椎病、上颈段椎骨错缝的治疗。

2. Pulling of the neck by supporting jaw with forearm

The patient is in the sitting position.Standing behind the patient, the physician supports the patient's jaw with one forearm that goes round the neck,puts the homolataral hand on the opposite shoulder, and opens the first web of the other hand to support the patient's occiput.Then takes the forearm for lever, and the shoulder for fulcrum to draw the head upward, meanwhile the other hand keeps the neck and the head in the neutral position(Fig. 264).It is allowed to make sudden and controlled shaking from left to right or from right to left so as to rotate the neck in narrow range.This manipulation is suitable for the treatments of cervical spondylopathy and upper cervical vertebral subluxation.

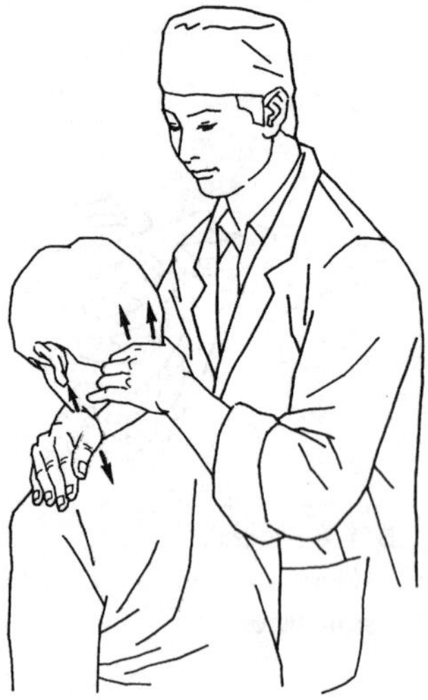

图264 前臂托颌拔颈法
Fig.264 Pulling of the neck by supporting jaw with forearm

3. 卧位拔颈法

患者仰卧，双手抓住两侧床沿。操作者以一手掌心托住患者下颌，另一手掌托住患者枕部，然后将其向后上方与水平线成30°角纵向牵拉(图265)。牵拉过程中可配合颈椎小幅度的屈伸、旋转、侧屈运动。本法适用于颈椎病、落枕的治疗。

3. Pulling of the neck in supine position

Lying in the supine position, the patient grasps two edges of the bed with hands. The physician holds the patient's jaw and occiput with his hand to pull the neck posteriosuperiorly at a direction of 30° with the horizontalline (Fig.265). It is allowed to coordinate with narrow ranged movements of flexion-extension, rotation and lateral bending of the neck during the pulling course. This manipulation is suitable for the treatments of cervi-

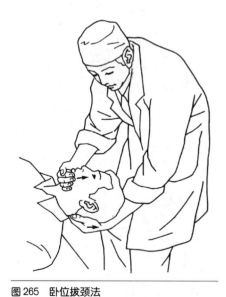

图265 卧位拔颈法
Fig. 265 Puling of the neck in supine position

cal spondy lopathy and stiff neck.

二、拔伸上肢
Pulling of Upper Limb

1. 夹腕拔肩法
患者坐位。操作者站于其患侧，用两膝内侧夹住患者腕部，使患肢远端固定；双手握住腋下，沿肱骨纵轴方向向上端拔伸（图266）。本法适用于肩周炎粘连期、陈旧性肩关节脱位的治疗。

1. Pulling shoulder while clipping wrist
The patient is in the sitting position. Standing on the suffered side, the physician clips the wrist with two medial sides of the knees to fix the distal portion of the limb and holds the armpit region with two hands to pull the shoulder upward along the long axis of the humerus (Fig.266). This manipulation is suitable for the treatments of the scapulohumeral periarthritis in the adhesion period and old dislocation of the scapulohumeral joint.

2. 膝顶拔肩法
患者坐位。操作者双手握紧其上臂下端，将一侧屈曲之膝部抵住患肩腋下，使身体稳定，然后两手后拉，膝部前顶，将患肢向远端牵拉（图267）。适应证同上。

2. Pulling shoulder while supporting armpit with knee
The patient is in the sitting position. The physician holds the distal end of the arm with hands, and puts a flexed knee to counterwork against the armpit of the suffered shoulder to fix the patient's body. With the hands and the knee energized to the contrary directions, draws the suffered shoulder (Fig.267). The indication of this manipulation is the same as above one.

3. 肩顶拔肩法
患者与操作者并排站立，操作者一侧上肢自后向前搂住患者腰部，肩部则顶住患者腋下，将患肢自操作者颈后垂下，用另一手握住其腕部，然后利用身体向前扭转之力，把患肩牵拉（图268）。本法利用腰胯力量拔伸肩关节，操作者较为省力，适用于陈旧性肩关节脱位的治疗。

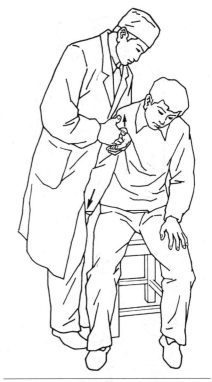

图266 夹腕拔肩法
Fig. 266 Pulling shoulder while clipping wrist

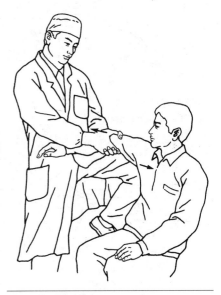

图267 膝顶拔肩法
Fig. 267 pulling shoulder while supporting armpit with knee

3. Pulling shoulder while supporting armpit with shoulder

The patient and the physician stand side by side. The physician hugs the patient's loins with an arm from back to front, bears against the patient's armpit with his shoulder to lets the suffered arm hang behind the physician's neck, and holds the wrist with the other hand, Then pulls the suffered shoulder by the means of trunk rotation forward (Fig.268). Because this manipulation makes use of the power of the loins and the pelvis, it is labor saving. It is suitable for the treatment of old dislocation of the scapulohumeral joint.

4. 腕关节拔伸法

操作者一手握住患者前臂下端，另一手握住其手，两手相对用力，将腕关节纵向牵拉(图269)。本法适用于腕关节扭伤的治疗。

4. Pulling of wrist

The physician holds the distal portion of the patient's forearm with one hand and holds the patient's hand with the other hand. With the two hands delivering force oppositely, pulls the wrist for a moment (Fig.269). This manipulation is suitable for the treatment of the sprain of the wrist joint.

5. 指间关节拔伸法

操作者以一手握住患手，另一手示、中指屈曲，夹住患指，两手相对用力，将手指纵向拔伸(图270)。本法适用于指间关节扭伤、扳机指的治疗。

5. Pulling of interphalangeal joint

The physician holds suffered hand with one hand and clips the suffered finger with the flexed index and middle finger of the other hand. With two hands delivering force oppositely, pulls the finger for a moment (Fig.270). This manipulation is suitable for the sprain of the interphalangeal joint and trigger finger.

三、拔伸躯干
Pulling of Trunk

患者俯卧位，两手抓住头端床沿。助手抓住患者两腋部，身

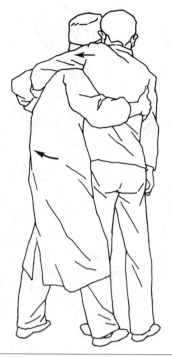

图268 肩顶拔肩法
Fig. 268 Pullillg shoulder while supporting armpit with shoulder

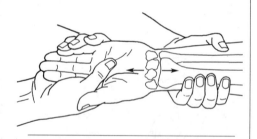

图269 腕关节拔伸法
Fig. 269 Pulling of wrist

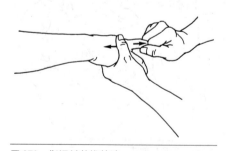

图270 指间关节拔伸法
Fig. 270 Pulling of interphalangeal joint

体后倾,作对抗用力。操作者以两腋夹住患者两足踝部,两脚蹬住床腿,身体后倾,利用足蹬和躯干腰背肌力量,将患者下肢向远端牵引(图271)。本法适用于腰椎间盘突出症的诊断。若拔伸后患者坐骨神经痛减轻,可能为脱出椎间盘压迫所致。

The patient is in the prone position, grasps the rostral edge of the bed with his two hands. An assistant holds the patient's armpits and inclines his body backward to bear against the traction force. The physician clips the patient's two ankles with his armpits, treads against the legs of the bed and inclines his body backward to pull the patient's lower limbs with the force of the lower limbs and the trunk muscles (Fig.271). This manipulation is suitable for the diagnose of the protrusion of the lumbar intervertebral disc. If the patient feels the sciatica being relieved during the pulling course, it is very possible to be the compression caused by protruded intervertebral disc.

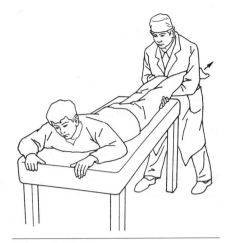

图271 拔伸躯干
Fig. 271 Pulling of trunk

四、拔伸下肢
Pulling of Lower Limb

1. 骶髂关节、髋关节拔伸法

患者仰卧,会阴部垫一软枕。操作者以一侧腋部夹住患肢足踝部,前臂从小腿后侧穿出,抓住另一侧以手握持患肢膝部的前臂,将患肢切实交锁住,用另一侧足蹬抵患者会阴部软枕;然后下肢前蹬,腰背后仰,利用躯干肌肉力量将患肢向远端牵引(图272)。本法适用于骶髂关节错缝、髋关节扭伤的治疗。

1. Pulling of sacroiliac joint and hip joint

The patient is in the supine position, with a soft cushion put under the patient's perineum. The physician clips the ankle of the suffered leg with his armpit and holds the knee with the contralateral hand and the homolateral forearm, while his homolateral hand passing behind the suffered leg and grasps himself's wrist of contraside. Then takes a foot to tread against the cushion and extends the spine to pull the lower limb backward with the force of the trunk muscles (Fig.272). This manipulation is suitable for the treatments of the subluxation of the sacroiliac

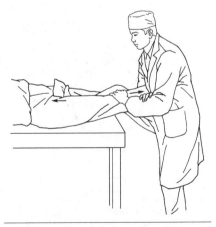

图272 骶髂关节、髋关节拔伸法
Fig. 272 Pulling of sacroiliac joint and hip joint

joint and the sprain of the hip joint.

2. 踝关节拔伸法

患者仰卧。操作者一手托患足跟部，另一手握跖趾部，沿胫骨纵轴方向向远端牵拉（图273）。本法适用于踝关节扭伤的治疗。

2. Pulling of ankle joint

The patient is in the supine position. The physician supports the suffered heel with one hand and holds the instep and toes with the other hand to pull the foot along the long axis of the tibia bone (Fig.273). This manipulation is suitable for the treatment of the sprain of the ankle joint.

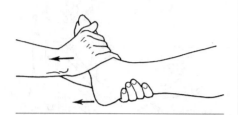

图273　踝关节拔伸法
Fig. 273　Pulling of ankle joint

第十三节　端提类手法
SECTION 13 CATEGORY OF LIFTING MANIPULATIONS

所谓端提类手法是指操作者握持患者肢体远端作一短促突发的向上用力，利用患者重力和静止惯性力稳定肢体近端而产生关节相对分离运动的一类手法操作。与拔伸类手法相比较，端提类手法虽然也沿肢体纵轴用力，但其作用过程十分短暂，而拔伸类手法则是持续用力。端提类手法可用图274模拟表示。

The so-called category of lifting manipulations means those actions in which the distal part of the patient's body or limb is held by the the physician while proximal part is kept in steady by the body weight and static inertial force. And then a brief and sudden lifting motion is done. Thus the joint facets is separated. Compared with the category of pulling-streching manipulations, a brief action is done in the former while constant force is delivered in the later. Though the two categories both use the force at the longitudinal axis of the body, their

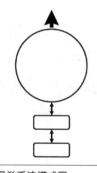

图274　端提类手法模式图
Fig. 274　Model of category of lifting Manipulations

acting courses are different. The category of lifting manipulations can be modeled with the Fig.274.

一、端提头颈
Lifting of Neck

1. 背后操作
　　患者坐位。操作者站于其身后，以两手掌托住其两侧下颌角下缘，并将患者枕部靠住自己胸前，把患者头部向后上方端提至限制位；适时作一突发动作，利用手与躯干的力量，扩大头颈运动幅度0.5 cm左右，随即放松(图275)。本法可使颈椎关节分离，利用肌肉和韧带的弹性力，促使错位交锁关节复位，本法适用于颈椎错缝而伴有前斜角肌痉挛患者的治疗。

1. Lifting of neck manipulated behind patient
　　The patient is in the sitting position. Standing behind the patient, the physician supports two lower rims of jaw with hands and puts the patient's occiput against the chest to lift the patient's head directed posterio-superiorly to the barrier position. Then makes a sudden action to extend the movement range of head and neck about half centimeter with the force produced by the hands and the trunk. Loosens the head immediately (Fig.275). This manipulation can separate the facets of cervical vertebral joints and restore the locked subluxation joint by means of the spring force of muscles and tendons. This manipulation is adapted to treat those subluxation sufferers who are complicated with the spasm of musculi scalenus anterior.

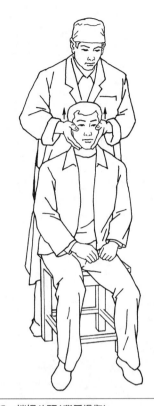

图275　端提头颈（背后操作）
Fig. 275　Lifting of neck (manipulated behind patient)

2. 前面操作
　　患者坐位。操作者站于其面前，两手虎口张开，托住下颌角和枕骨下缘，以屈曲的手指指间关节顶住错位前凸之颈椎横突前结节；两手协同用力，将头部向上端提并作小幅度左右摇晃，以放松颈肌；适时作一突发有控制的端提动作，向患者后上方用力，同时手指顶推颈椎横突，使其复位(图276)。本法适用于颈椎错缝伴有前斜角肌痉挛患者的治疗。

2. Lifting of neck manipulated in front of patient
　　The patient is in the sitting position. Standing in front of the patient, the physician supports two mandibulae

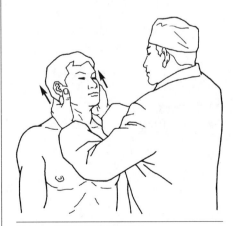

图276　端提头颈（前面操作）
Fig.276　Lifting of neck (manipulated in front of patient)

and the lower rims of the occiput with his opened first webs of both hands, and contacts against the projected anterior tubercle of the transverse process of the suffered segment with his flexed interphalangeal joints. Then pulls the head up and makes narrow ranged shaking left to right to relax cervical muscles by the means of two hands acting coordinately. Then makes a sudden and controlled lifting directed posterio-superiorly. At this moment, thrusts the transverse process at the same time to restore the subluxation (Fig.276). This manipulation is also adapted to treat those cervical vertebral subluxation sufferers who are complicated with the spasm of the musculi scalenus anterior.

二、端提胸胁
Lifting of Thorax and Ribs

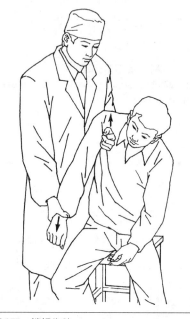

图277 端提胸胁
Fig. 277 Lifting of thorax and ribs

患者坐位。操作者站于其患侧，以一侧上肢前臂从患侧腋下穿过，屈肘，上提肩部，另一手握其腕部以稳定患侧上肢；然后嘱患者深呼吸，每当吸气终了时上提患肩并随即放松，连续数次；待患者呼吸自然，肌肉放松时，乘某一吸气期末，适时用力迅速上提患肩，即可听到复位声。本法适用于胸6节段以上肋椎关节错缝的治疗（图277）。

The patient is in the sitting position. Standing on the suffered side, the physician lifts the shoulder with flexed elbow that is inserted through the armpit, and holds the patient's wrist with the other hand to steady the upper limb. Then asks the patient to take deep breath. At the end of one inhalation period, lifts the suffered shoulder up and loosens it immediately. A restoration sound can be heard. This manipulation is adapted to treat the costovertebral joint subluxation that is above the T6 (Fig.277).

三、端提腰椎
Lifting of Lumbar Vertebrae

患者坐位。操作者站于其身后，两手从患者腋下伸过，环抱患者胸部，使患者腰部作小幅度左右旋转、摇晃和屈伸运动，待患者动作配合，肌肉放松时，适时将患者身体向后上方端提起，常可听到复位声(图278)。本法适用于伴有腰椎生理前凸增大、腰椎假性滑脱等情况的腰椎错缝者的治疗。

The patient is in the sitting position. Standing behind the patient, the physician inserts two hands through the armpits to hug the patient's chest roundly. Then makes the patient's waist be rotated and shaked left to right, flexed to extended. As the patient's action is coordinated and his muscles relaxed, lifts the body briefly and directed posterio-superiorly at the very time. A restoration sound can be heard (Fig.278). This manipulation is suitable for the treatments of those patients who are suffered from subluxation of the lumbar vertebrae complicated with increased physiological curve of the lumbar vertebrae or pseudo lumbar spondylolisthesis.

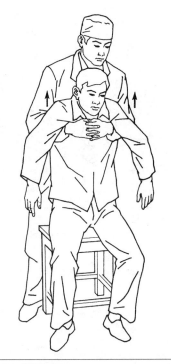

图278 端提腰椎
Fig. 278 Lifting of lumbar vertebrae

第十四节　抖动类手法
SECTION 14 CATEGORY OF SHAKING MANIPULATIONS

所谓抖动类手法是指操作者持患者肢体一端进行上下小幅度抖动，使肢体组织产生纵波振动，并将这一振动传递到远处的一类操作。抖动类手法可用图279模拟表示。

The so-called "category of shaking manipulations" means those actions in which the physician holds the distal part of the limb and shakes it up and downward in narrow range, so as to cause the limb to be vibrated longitudlnally and take this vibration to transmit to proximal of the limb. This category of shaking manipulation can be modeled with Fig.279.

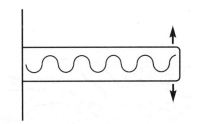

图279 抖动类手法模式图
Fig. 279 Model of category of shaking manipulations

一、抖上肢
Shaking of Upper Limb

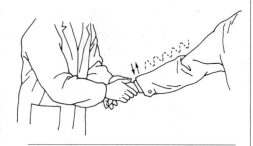

图 280 抖上肢
Fig. 280 Shaking of upper limb

患者坐位，肩部放松，上肢下垂。操作者站于其前外侧，双手并握患肢前臂下端，在患肩外展、前屈45°位下微用力作小幅度的上下连续抖动，幅度由大渐小，频率由低而高，使振动由腕部逐渐传达到肩部，整个上肢产生明显的舒松感(图280)。本法具有疏通经脉，松解筋肉，滑利关节的作用，常用作治疗肩、肘关节疼痛、运动障碍的结束手法。

The patient is in the sitting position, relaxes his shoulder and drops his upper limb. Standing on the anteriolateral side of the patient, the physician holds the lower end of the suffered arm with two hands. Then shakes the upper limb up and downward in narrow range gently, while the shoulder joint is kept in 45° of abduction and flexion. The range of shaking is changed from broader to narrower while the frequency changed from lower to higher. The manipulator should make the vibration transmit to the shoulder gradually and the whole upper limb produce a relaxed and comfortable feeling(Fig.280). This manipulation possesses the functions of dredging blocked channels and vessels, relaxing muscles and loosening tendons, as well as lubricating the joint. It is usually used to treat pain and motion obstacle in the shoulder and elbow joints, as the final manipulation.

二、抖腕部
Shaking of Wrist

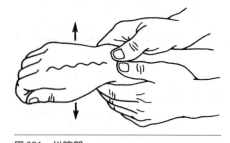

图 281 抖腕部
Fig. 281 Shaking of wrist

操作者双手自上而下并握前臂下端，作小幅度上下连续抖动，使腕手自由地连续震抖。本法适用于治疗腕关节疼痛、活动不利，常作为结束手法使用(图281)。

The physician holds the patient's lower end of forearm with two hands and makes continually shaking in narrow range. This manipulation is suitable for the treatment of pain and inconvenient motion in the wrist joint, usually as a final manipulation(Fig.281).

三、抖下肢
Shaking of Lower Limb

患者仰卧。操作者站于其足端，两手并握踝部，在下肢伸直抬高30°位置下将其踝部作小幅度的上下连续颤抖，幅度由大到小，频率由慢到快，但一般要比抖上肢时慢，前者的频率为每分钟200～240次，本法频率为每分钟140～160次。本法适用于髋、膝关节疼痛、功能障碍的治疗，常作为结束手法使用(图282)。

The patient is in the supine position. Standing on the foot side, the physician holds the ankle of suffered limb and keeps the leg in straight and the hip flexed to 30°. Then shakes the ankle up and downward. The range of shaking is varied from broader to narrower while the frequency varied from lower to higher. But in general, it is slower than shaking of upper limb. The frequency of the former is about 200 to 240 times a minute, while the frequency of this manipulation is about 140 to 160 times a minute. The manipulation is adapted to the treatments of pain and motion obstacle in the hip and knee joints. It is used as a final manipulation (Fig.282).

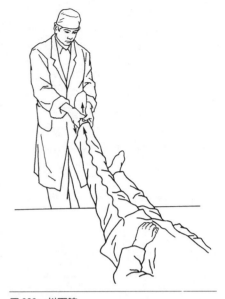

图282 抖下肢
Fig. 282 Shaking of lower limb

四、抖腰
Shaking of Waist

患者俯卧，双手用力抓住床头。操作者以一侧腋下夹住患者两踝部，脚尖抵住床脚，身体后仰，将患者下肢在后伸位下向远端牵拉片刻；然后在保持拔伸作用下左右摇动患者下肢，待患者腰部放松时，突然上下抖动下肢；再用力牵拉，重复操作数次(图283)。本法具有解除腰椎后关节滑膜嵌顿，放松腰肌张力，促进椎间盘突出物移位回纳的作用，用于急性腰扭伤、腰椎错缝、腰椎间盘突出症的治疗。

The patient is in the prone position. The physician clips the patient's ankles with armpit, treads against the bed legs with the toes and inclines his body backward to pull the lower limb distally by the means of extending his trunk for a moment. Then shakes the lower limbs left to right under traction. As the patient's lumbar is being relaxed, suddenly shakes the lower limbs up and

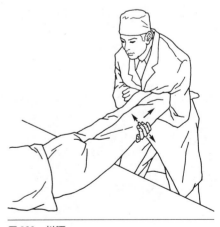

图283 抖腰
Fig.283 Shaking of waist

downward. And then pulls the lower limbs again. Repeats these manipulation several times (Fig.283). This manipulation can remove the strapped synovialis in the posterior joint of the lumbar vertebrae, loosen the tension of lumbar muscles and promote the prorupted nuclear to move away or to revert. It is used for the treatments of acute sprain of the lumbar, subluxation of the lumbar vertebra and protrusion of lumbar intervertebral disc.

第三章 推拿操作常规

CHAPTER 3 THE ROUTINE TECHNIQUES OF TUINA

一、头面部操作常规
The Routine Techniques on Head and Facial Regions

1. 体位
坐位。
1. Position
Sitting.

2. 重点刺激穴位
睛明、太阳、下关、颊车、鱼腰、头维、角孙、风池、桥弓。
2. Key points of stimulation
Jingming(BL 1), Taiyang(EX-HN5), Xiaguan (ST7), Jiache(ST6), Yuyao(EX-HN4), Touwei(ST8), Jiaosun (TE20), Fengchi (GB20), Qiaogong(Tuina point).

3. 主要手法
一指禅推、抹、按揉、拿、拇指平推。
3. Main manipulations
Dhyana-thumb pushing, wiping, pressing-kneading grasping and flat pushing with thumb.

4. 操作步骤
(1)以一指禅偏峰推法推面部，其具体路线是：从印堂穴起沿额部正中线至神庭，沿发际缘推到头维，折向下方抵太阳穴，左右两侧各往返数次(图284)。当推到头维穴处，由于额角处平面发生转折，初学者常会产生指端滑脱，可调整手的空间位置，使拇指纵轴与移动路线平行，能改善拇指吸附能力。

再从印堂出发，沿眼眶内缘作"∞"字形移动，即推上眼眶时自目内眦推向目外眦，推下眼眶时自目外眦推向目内眦(图285)。推眼眶时，手腕摆动幅度要小，移动宜缓慢，以防止拇指滑脱而戳碰眼球。但推至目内眦经鼻梁骨到另侧目内眦过程中，由于骨面崎岖不平坦，亦易滑脱。操作时可略改变方向，先从目内眦推至印堂穴，再从印堂穴移至另侧目内眦，就较容易操作。最后，从印堂出发，沿鼻梁外侧、颧弓下缘推至下关穴，沿下颌骨下颌支推到颊车，折向内移动至地仓穴后再环绕口轮匝肌一周，沿原线返回印堂，左右往返数次(图286)。推面颊部时，若患者肥胖，拇指将陷在皮肉内，难以移动，可一方面减轻压力，另一方面改变手的位置，使拇指纵轴与移动路线垂直，就容易操作。

4. Manipulation steps

The first step, the manipulation Dhyana-thumb pushing is manipulated on the face. The moving routes of the thumb are as below: From the point Yintang to the point Shenting(GV24) along the middle line of forehead, then along the anterior hairline to the point Touwei, then turning down to the point Taiyang, then going back along the same way. The above manipulation is repeated for a few times in the right and left side respectively (Fig.284). When the thumb is moving at the point Touwei, due to the uneven surface, the learner often slips his thumb tip away. If one adjusts the hand location in the space to make the long axis of the thumb in paralled line with the moving route, the attraction ability of the thumb may be enhanced. Latter, from the point Yintang to Yintang along the inner rims of the eye sockets as a "∞" mark, i.e. moving on the upper rim, the direction is from the medial angle of the eye to lateral angle, while moving on the lower rim, the direction is from lateral to medial (Fig.285). When moving on inner rim of the eye socket, the swinging range of wrist should be reduced and the moving speed should be decelerated in order to avoid the thumb slipping and hurting the eye ball. Even that, it is also easy for the thumb to be slipped when moving from the inner angle of one eye through the nose bridge to the other, due to the bone surface is rugged. It can be avoided in this way, manipulating from the inner angle to the point Yintang, then from which

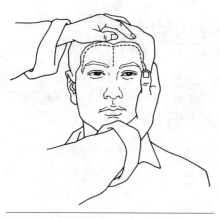

图284 一指禅推额部
Fig. 284 Dhyana-thumb pushing on forehead

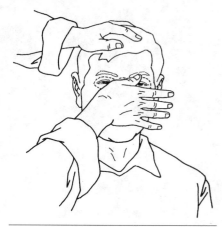

图285 一指禅推眼眶
Fig. 285 Dhyana-thumb pushing on eye sockets

to the other inner angle. Finally, from the point Yintang along the lateral side of nose, the lower rim of the cheekbone to the point Xiaguan, and along the jaw bone to the point Jiache, then turning medially to the point Dicang, then moving around the mouth and returning to the point Yintang along the same routes. The moving route is stimulated for several times in both sides respectively (Fig.286). If the patient is fatty, as moving on the cheek region, the thumb will be sunk in the flesh and be difficult to move about. It will be easy to manipulate in this way, which is reducing the pressing force and changing the hand position to make the long axis of the thumb in vertical to the moving route.

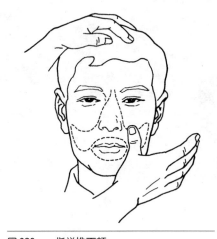

图286 一指禅推面颊
Fig. 286 Dhyana-thumb pushing on face

(2)沿上述路线用抹法,并在抹的过程中自然配合点揉睛明、鱼腰、太阳、头维、角孙、下关、颊车等穴(图46)。

The second step, the wiping is exerted on the same route as above and is naturally coordinated with kneading at the point Jingming, Yuyao, Taiyang, Touwei, Jiaosun, Xiaguan, Jiache(Fig.46)

(3)用拇指平推法自上而下推桥弓,每侧15次(图287)。

The third step, the manipulation, flat pushing with thumb, is applied along the linear point Qiaogong up to down and repeated for 15 times in right and left side respectively (Fig.287).

(4)用扫散法在颞部胆经区域操作,每侧各15次。

The fourth step, the sweeping is manipulated on the region of the Gallbladder Channel in the temple portion for 15 times in each side.

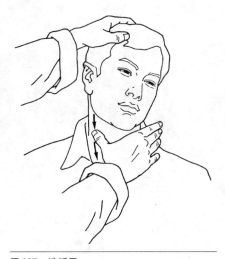

图287 推桥弓
Fig. 287 Pushing on Qiaogong

(5)抓头顶,抓时五指分开,中指对准督脉,示指、环指对准两侧膀胱经,拇指、小指对准两侧胆经,边抓边移向枕部;至枕部后改为三指拿,拿风池、拿项部肌肉、拿两侧肩井,结束操作。

The fifth step, the routine is ended with seizing in this way. The manipulator opens the fingers, seizes the head and gradually moves stimulation point to the occiput while seizing, with the middle finger on the Du

Channel, the index and the ring fingers on the Urinary Bladder Channel of Foot Taiyang, and the thumb and the little finger on the Gallbladder Channel of Foot Shaoyang. After that, the manipulation is substituted by grasping at the point Fengchi, on the muscles of the nape and at the point Jianjing(GB21).

5. 适应证

凡头痛、失眠、高血压、感冒、面瘫、三叉神经痛等病证均可用头面部操作常规作为基本操作程序,并根据辨证、辨病论治,予以增减。

5. Indications

Headache, insomnia, cold, hypertension, facial paralysis and trigeminal neuralgia can be treated with this routine on head and face as their basic therapeutically program, which is allowed to be modified according to different syndromes and disorders.

二、颈项部操作常规
The Routine Techniques on Neck and Nape Regions

1. 体位

坐位。

1. Position

Sitting.

2. 重点刺激穴位

风池、夹脊、肩井、扶突、肩中俞、天宗。

2. Key points of stimulation

Fengchi(GB 20), Jiaji(EX-B2), Jianjing (GB 21), Futu (LI 18), Jianzhongshu(SI 15) and Tianzong(SI 11).

3. 主要手法

滚法、一指禅推法、拿法、按揉法、环摇、推扳法。

3. Main manipulations

Rolling, Dhyana-thumb pushing, grasping, pressing-kneading, rotating and thrusting-wrenching.

4. 操作步骤

(1)先以一指禅偏峰推两手同时操作,刺激风池穴(蝴蝶双飞)1分钟(见图79),再以双手交叉扶持推两侧颈部,沿夹脊穴路线,自风府旁至定喘,上下往返数次。

4. Manipulation steps

The first step, dhyana-thumb pushing is applied to stimulate the point Fengchi on both sides simultaneously (couple flying butterflies) for one minute (Fig.79). Then the dhyana-thumb pushing supported by two crossed hands is followed on both sides of the cervical vertebrae from the point Fengfu to the point Dingchuan to and fro. for several times.

(2)先㨰颈项部及肩背部,自枕下至肩胛骨内侧缘间区,以放松肌肉,再边㨰颈项,边配合颈椎俯仰旋转侧屈扳动,约5分钟(参见图179~182)。

The second step, rolling on the cervix, shoulder and back regions, up to the subocciput and down to the interval of the medial rims of the scapulae to relax the muscles; coordinated the rolling with the flexion, extension, rotation, lateral flexion wrenching of the neck for 5 minute(look at Fig.179 to Fig.182).

(3)拿风池、拿项肌、拿肩井。

The third step, Grasping is applied at the point Fengchi, on the nape muscle and at the point Jianjing.

(4)点揉风池、肩井、扶突、天宗、肩中俞。

The fourth step, pressing kneading is applied at the points Fengchi, Jianjing, Futu, Tianzong, and Jianzhongshu.

(5)根据辨证、辨病论治原则,选用合适的颈椎复位手法。

The fifth step, reduction of the cervical vertebrae (selected step). Based on the principles of "treatment in accordance with overall analysis of symptoms and signs" as well as "treatment in accordance with overall analysis of pathological mechanisms", some suitable reduction of the cervical vertebrae are done.

(6)滚颈项、滚肩背。

The sixth step, rolling. It is manipulated on the cervical, shoulder and back regions again.

(7)摇颈。

The seventh step, rotating of neck.

5. 适应证

凡落枕、颈椎病、前斜角肌综合征，均可选用颈项部操作常规为基本操作程序，并予手法增减。

5. Indications

All the stiff neck, cervical spondylopathy and syndrome of the musculi scalenus anterior can be treated with the routine, which could be modified if necessary.

三、肩部操作常规

The Routine Techniques on the Shoulder Region

1. 体位

坐位或卧位。

1. Position

setting or lying.

2. 重点刺激穴位

肩髃、肩内陵、天鼎、缺盆、外天宗、尺泽、曲池、合谷、外关。

2. Key points of stimulation

Jianyu (LI 15), Jianneiling (Extra), Tianding (LI 17), Quepen (ST 12), Waitianzong (Extra), Chize (LU 5), Quchi (LI 11), Hegu (LI 4) and Waiguan (TE 15).

3. 主要手法

滚法、一指禅推法、拿法、按揉法、环摇、推扳、搓法、抖动。

3. Main manipulations

Rolling, dhyana-thumb pushing, grasping, pressing-kneading, rotating, thrusting-wrenching, rubbing with two palms and shaking.

4. 操作步骤

(1)㨰颈项、肩背部,以放松斜方肌、肩胛提肌、菱形肌。

4. Manipulation steps

The first step, rolling. The manipulation is delivered on the cervical and upper back regions to relax the trapezius, levator scapulae and rhomboideus.

(2)一指禅推天鼎、缺盆穴,使手法感应传导至肩痛部位(图288)。然后用一指禅推肩内陵、肩髃穴。

The second step, dhyana-thumb pushing. The manipulation is applied at the points Tianding and Quepen to make the manipulative feeling be transmitted to the painful portion of the shoulder(Fig.288),then at the point Jianneiling and the point Jianyu.

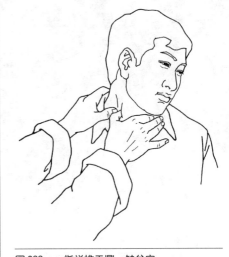

图 288 一指禅推天鼎、缺盆穴
Fig. 288 Dhyana-thumb pushing on points Tianding and Quepen

(3)㨰肩关节周围,配合肩关节外展、前举、内收、旋转、后弯(参见图188~198)。㨰肘窝,配合肘关节伸展、前臂外旋扳动(图289),以消除肱二头肌下端止点的损伤性炎症。

The third step, rolling. The manipulation is delivered on the surrounding regions of the shoulder coordinated with the manipulation of abduction-wrench, flexion-wrenching, adduction-wrenching, rotation-wrenching and posterior bending-wrenching of the shoulder(look at the Fig.188 to Fig.198). The elbow hollow is stimulated with rolling and coordinated with the extension wrenching of elbow and supination-wrenching of forearm to remove inflammation due to injury at the lower attaching point of the biceps brachia(Fig.289).

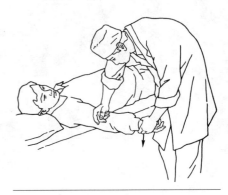

图 289 㨰肘窝配合肘关节运动
Fig. 289 Rolling on elbow hollow coordinated with extension wrenching of elbow

(4)拿揉肩关节循臂而下,重点刺激尺泽、曲池、手三里、合谷、外关,重复3次。

The fourth step, grasping-kneading. The upper limb is stimulated from the shoulder to the hand with the grasping-kneading, and focally stimulated at the points Chize, Quchi, Shousanli, Hegu and Waiguan, for three times.

(5)环摇肩关节。

The fifth step, rotating of shoulder.

(6)搓肩臂，抖上肢，结束操作。

The sixth step, The routine is finished with the manipulation rubbing with two palms on shoulder, arm and hand, and then shaking of upper limb.

5. 适应证

凡肩关节周围炎、肩袖病、肱二头肌长头腱鞘炎均可以肩部操作常规为基本操作程序，并根据其病理特点而增减。

5. Indications

All the scapulohumeral periarthritis, shoulder-rotator cuff disease and tendinous synovitis of the long head of biceps can be treated with this routine, which can be modified depending on the pathological characters of the patients.

四、肘部操作常规
The Routine Techniques on the Elbow Region

1. 体位

坐位或卧位。

1. Position

Sitting or lying.

2. 重点刺激穴位

曲池、手三里、尺泽、少海。

2. Key points of stimulation

Quchi(LI 11), Shousanli(LI 10), Chize(LU 5) and Shaohai (HT 3).

3. 主要手法

滚法、按法、弹拨、拿法、推扳、环摇、搓法。

3. Main manipulations

rolling, pressing, plucking, grasping, thrusting wrenching, rotating and rubbing with two palms.

4. 操作步骤

(1)先㨰肘关节周围及前臂约3分钟，以减轻疼痛，放松肌肉，便于操作。接着边㨰肘关节周围，边配合肘关节扳法；边㨰肘窝部，边配合肘关节伸展扳动(图289)；边㨰肘后部，边配

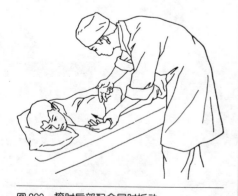

图290 㨰肘后部配合屈肘扳动
Fig. 290 Rolling on the posterior region coordinated with flexion-wrenching of elbow

合肘关节屈曲扳动(圆290)；边搽肘关节桡侧，边配合前臂旋前及屈腕扳动(图291)；边搽肘关节内侧，边配合前臂旋后及伸腕扳动(图292)。

4. Manipulation steps

The first step, rolling and thrusting-wrenching. The manipulation, rolling, is exerted on the surrounding regions of the elbow and the forearm for 3 minutes, so as to relieve pain, relax muscles and facilitate later manipulation. Then it is coordinated with wrenching of elbow as follows: Rolling on the elbow hollow and coordinated with extension-wrenching of elbow(Fig.289), rolling on the posterior part of elbow and coordinated with flexion-wrenching of elbow(Fig.290), rolling on the radial side of elbow and coordinated with the pronation-wrenching of forearm and flexion-wrenching of wrist (Fig.291), rolling on the ulnar side of elbow and coordinated with supination-wrenching of forearm and extension-wrenching of wrist (Fig.292).

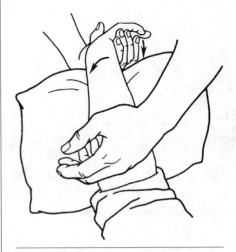

图291 搽肘桡侧配合旋前屈腕扳动
Fig. 291 Rolling on the radial region of elbow coordinated with the pronation-wrenching of forearm and flexion-wrenching of wrist

(2)拿揉前臂，循肘关节而下，重点刺激曲池、尺泽、手三里、少海、外关、合谷穴。

The second step, grasping-kneading. Stimulation is applied on the forearm from the elbow to the wrist with the manipulation grasping-kneading. The key points of stimulation are Quchi, Chize, Shousanli, Shaohai, Waiguan and Hegu.

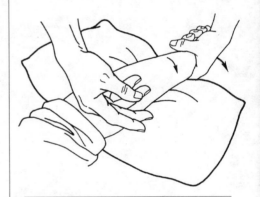

图292 搽肘尺侧配合旋后伸腕扳动
Fig. 292 Rolling on ulnar region of elbow coordinated with wrenching of supination and wrist extension

(3)用拇指弹拨肘部压痛点，以分离粘连。

The third step, plucking. Plucking with the thumb is done at the trigger point of the elbow region to split away the adhesion.

(4)摇肘关节。

The fourth step, rotating of elbow.

(5)擦热压痛点局部。

The fifth step, linear rubbing. The manipulation linear rubbing with the thenar is delivered at the trigger point of the elbow to warm the deep tissues.

(6)搓肘部、前臂，结束治疗。

The sixth step, rubbing with two palms. The manipulation is exerted on the elbow and the forearm to finish the routine.

5. 适应证

凡肘关节扭伤、肘关节周围粘连、网球肘、高尔夫球肘、矿工肘均可用肘部操作常规为基本操作程序，予以增减。

5. Indications

All the sprain of the elbow, periarthral adhesion of the elbow, tennis elbow, golf elbow and miner elbow can be treated with this manipulation routine, which can be modified depending on the symptoms and disorders of the patients.

五、腕手操作常规
The Routine Techniques on the Wrist and the Hand Regions

1. 体位

坐位。

1. Position

Sitting.

2. 重点刺激穴位

内关、外关、大陵、合谷、阳溪。

2. Key points of stimulation

Neiguan(PC 6), Waiguan(TE 5), Daling(PC 7), Hegu(LI 4) and Yangxi(LI 5).

3. 主要手法

滚、按揉、拿、捻、环摇、推扳。

3. Main manipulations

rolling, pressing-kneading, grasping, holding-kneading, rotating and thrusting-wrenching.

4. 操作步骤

(1)先滚前臂及腕关节周围，以减轻局部疼痛，放松肌肉。然后拔伸腕关节(或指间关节)，再边滚腕部，边配合腕关节扳法。

其方法为：边搓腕关节桡侧，边配合腕关节尺偏扳动(图293)；边搓腕掌侧，边配合腕背伸扳动(图294)；边搓腕尺侧，边配合腕桡偏扳动；边搓腕背侧，边配合腕掌屈扳动。

4. Manipulation steps

The first step, rolling and thrusting-wrenching. The rolling manipulation is employed on the forearm and wrist region to relieve local pain and relax muscles, then pulling of the wrist is followed and then the rolling coordinated with wrenching of wrist is succeeded in this way: Rolling on the radial side of the wrist and coordinated with adduction-wrenching of wrist(Fig.293), rolling on the palm side of the wrist and coordinated with extension-wrenching of the wrist (Fig.294), rolling on the ulnar side of the wrist and coordinated with the abduction-wrenching of the wrist, rolling on the back side of the wrist and coordinated with the flexion-wrenching of the wrist.

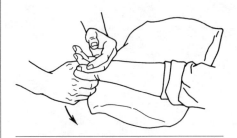

图293 滚腕桡侧配合尺屈扳
Fig. 293 Rolling on radial side of wrist coordinated with adduction-wrenching

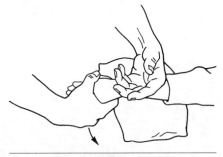

图294 滚腕掌侧配合伸腕扳
Fig. 294 Rolling on palm side of wrist coordinated with extension-wrenching

(2)拿揉前臂、腕部、手掌，重点刺激内关、外关、大陵、合谷、阳溪穴，捏各掌骨间隙，捻各指。

The second step, grasping-kneading. Stimulation is applied on the forearm from the elbow to the wrist with the manipulation grasp-kneading. The key points of manipulation are Neiguan, Waiguan, Daling, Hegu, and Yangxi. Then pinching is followed along all the intermetacarpal spaces, and holding-kneading succeded on all fingers and the thumb.

(3)摇腕部(或指关节)。

The third step, rotating of the wrist or rotating of the interphalangeal joint.

(4)擦热局部。

The fourth step, linear-rubbing. Linear-rubbing is delivered on the injured part to warm the deep tissue.

(5)搓、抖腕部，结束操作。

The fifth step, the rubbing with two palms and shaking are employed on the wrist to finish treatment.

5. 适应证

凡腕关节扭伤、下尺桡关节损伤、狭窄性腱鞘炎、腕管综合征均可以腕手操作常规为基本操作程序，予以增减。

5. Indications

All the sprain of the wrist, injury of the inferior radial—ulnar joint, stenosal tendovaginitis and carpal tunnel syndrome can be treated with this routine, which can be modified.

六、腰背部操作常规
The Routine Techniques on the Back Region

1. 体位
俯卧位。
1. Position
Pronation.

2. 重点刺激穴位
夹脊、肺俞、心俞、肝俞、脾俞、胃俞、肾俞、腰眼、髂腰角、臀上皮神经区。
2. Key points of Stimulation
Jiaji (EX−B2), Feishu(BL 13), Xinshu(BL 15), Ganshu (BL 18), Pishu(BL 20), Weishu(BL 21), Shenshu(BL 23), Yaoyan(EX−B7), iliolumbar angle, region of the nervi clunis superiors.

3. 主要手法
滚、按、弹拨、推扳、环摇。
3. Main manipulations
rolling, pressing, plucking, thrusting−wrenching and rotating.

4. 操作步骤
（1）先在脊柱两侧用滚法操作，自上而下，自下面上，往返数遍，左右交替，以放松骶棘肌。滚法操作过程中应避免掌指关节骨突撞击棘突，引起疼痛不适。
4. Manipulation steps
The first step, rolling. The rolling manipulation is delivered on both sides of the spine up and down and

alternately on right and left side for several times, so that the sacrospinalis muscle is relaxed. One should avoid the bone bulges of the metacarpal-phalangeal joints hitting the spinal processes and causing pain and uncomfortable.

(2)以拇指按压有关夹脊、背俞及背部筋结反应点，再用掌按法循脊柱自上而下轻压胸腰椎棘突，注意呼气时按脊，吸气时移动。按压过程中常可闻及弹响声，以纠正椎骨细微错移(图295)。

The second step, pressing. Pressing with the thumb is delivered on the relevant points Jiaji, Beishu, and trigger points where entangled nodules are palpated. Then the pressing with the palms is manipulated gently on the spine up downward. Pay attention on that the pressing is given in exhalation while moving to another segment in inhalation. During the pressing course, a spring sound, which indicates little shift of vertebrae is restored, may often be heard (Fig.295).

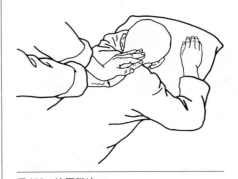

图295 按压脊柱
Fig. 295 Pressing on spine

(3) 㨰两腰部，边㨰边配合下肢后伸扳动(参见图223)。

The third step, rolling coordinated with the wrenching. The rolling is applied on both sides of the waist, meanwhile the wrenching of the lumbar vertebrae by extending lower extremity is coordinated (look at the Fig.223).

(4)以两手拇指相叠，按揉或弹拨腰2～4横突、骼腰角、臀上皮神经区，以刺激穴位，分离粘连，减轻疼痛(选择性)。

The fourth step, plucking(selected step). Two overlapped thumbs are employed to give the pressing-kneading or plucking on the transverse processes of the second lumbar vertebra to the fourth lumbar vertebra, the iliolumbar angle and the region of the nervi clunium superiors, so as to stimulate points, separate adhesion and relieve pain.

(5)根据疾病病理特点及节段高低，有选择地应用胸腰椎或肋椎关节复位手法(选择性)。

The fifth step, reduction of subluxation(Selected step). on the basis of the pathological characters and the level of the suffered segment, the manipulator can employ the corresponding reductions of the thoracic vertebrae, the lumbar vertebrae or the costovertebral joint.

(6)擦脊柱两侧。
The sixth step, rolling on both sides of the spine.

(7)擦两侧膀胱经，横擦损伤节段局部，搓腰部。
The seventh step, linear-rubbing.The linear-rubbing is done along the two Urinary Bladder Channels (vertical rubbing) and along the injured segment level (transverse rubbing). Then the rubbing with two palms is delivered on waist.

(8)仰卧、摇腰、顺时针方向及逆时针方向各摇15次。
The eighth step, rotating. The patient is in the supine position.The manipulator rotates the lumbar at both the clockwise direction and the anti-clockwise direction for 15 times.

5. 适应证
凡胸背软组织损伤、岔气、闪腰、腰椎间盘突出症、腰肌劳损等症均可用腰背操作常规为基本操作程序，并根据其病理特点予以增减。

5. Indications
All the soft tissue injuries of back,facet syndromes of the thoracic and lumbar vertebrae, subluxation of the costovertebral joint, sprain of the lumbar, protrusion of the lumbar intervertebral disc and the strain of the lumbar muscles can be treated with this routine, which can be modified according to the pathological characters.

七、胸腹部操作常规
The Routine Techniques on the Thoracoabdominal Regions

1. 体位
仰卧位。
1. Position
Supine.

2. 重点刺激穴位

膻中、中脘、天枢、关元、章门、期门、肺俞、心俞、肝俞、胆俞、脾俞、胃俞、肾俞、次髎。

2. Key points of stimulation

Tanzhong(CV 17), Zhongwan(CV 12), Tianshu (ST 25), Guanyuan(CV 4), Zhangmen(LR 13), Qimen(LR 14), Feishu(BL 13), Xinshu(BL 15), Ganshu(BL 18), Danshu (BL 19), Pishu(BL 20), Weishu(BL 21), Shenshu(BL 23), Ciliao(BL 32).

3. 主要手法

摩法、一指禅推、按揉、擦法。

3. Main manipulations

Round-rubbing, Dhyana-thumb pushing, Pressing kneading, Linear-rubbing.

4. 操作步骤

(1)先以拇指偏峰推胸部任脉路线、患处肋间隙，或用推摩法在腹部操作，配合点揉募穴，约10分钟。

4. Manipulation steps

The first step, dhyana-pushing with side tip of thumb. The Dhyana-pushing with side tip of thumb is done on the area along the Ren Channel and the suffered intercostal spaces. Or the Dhyana pushing and round-rubbing is manipulated on abdomen, coordinated with kneading on the Front-Mu points of the thoracoabdominal region. The step last for 10 minutes.

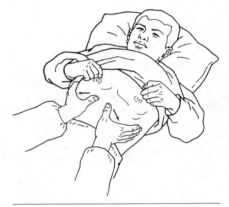

图296 分推腹部
Fig. 296 Eccentric-pushing on abdomen

(2)分推膻中或分推腹部，50～100次(图296)。

The second step, eccentric pushing on the Tanzhong or abdomen about 50 to 100 times (Fig.296).

(3)掌擦两胁肋或少腹，以微热为度(图297)。

The third step, the linear-rubbing is exerted on the two hypochondrium region or the two-hypogastric region until the patient fells slight warm into the manipulated area (Fig.297).

(4)俯卧，以一指禅推循两侧膀胱经在病变脏腑有关的背俞

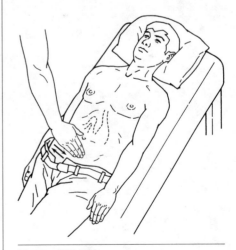

图297 掌擦少腹
Fig. 297 Linear-rubbing with palm on lower abdomen

穴上操作，上下往返数次，约5分钟。擦热膀胱经。

The fourth step, the patient is in the prone position. The Dhyana-thumb pushing is done at the points, which are concerned with the suffered viscera along the two Urinary Bladder Channels to and fro for 5 minutes. Then liner rubbing is manipulated on the distribution region along the Urinary Bladder Channel until the patient fells the deep tissues warmed.

(5)循经取穴，按揉有关十二经穴位。

The fifth step, the pressing-kneading is given at the relative points along the channel to stimulate the concerned points of the 12 Channels.

5. 适应证

凡胸腹腔内脏疾病，均可以胸腹部操作常规为基本操作法，再根据其病理特点予以增减。

5. Indications

All the visceral diseases in the thoracic and abdominal cavities can be treated with this routine, which can be modified depended on the pathological characters.

八、髋臀部操作常规
The Routine Techniques on the Buttock and the Hip Regions

1. 体位
卧位。
1. Position
Lying.

2. 重点刺激穴位
次髎、环跳、臀上皮神经区、腹股沟区、耻骨梳、臀中肌、阔筋膜张肌。
2. Key points of stimulation
Ciliao(UB32), Huantiao(GB30), Region of the nervi clunium superiors, groin, comb of pubis, gluteus medius and tensor fasciae latae.

3. 主要手法

滚法、按揉、弹拨、推扳。

3. Main manipulations

Rolling, Pressing-kneading, Plucking and Thrusting-wrenching.

4. 操作步骤

(1)俯卧。擦两侧腰部，配合下肢后伸扳动(参见图223)。

4. Manipulation steps

The first step, the patient lies in the prone position. Rolling is done on two sides of the waist and coordinated with the wrenching of lumbar by extending lower extremity (look at Fig.223).

(2)滚臀部、大腿后侧至腘窝部，上下往返3遍；再滚梨状肌体表区，配合髋内旋扳动(参见图240)。

The second step, rolling is done on the buttock, posterior side of the thigh and hollow of the knee to and fro for 3 times. Then while rolling on the surface region of the piriformis, the medial rotation-wrenching of the hip is done to coordinate the rolling manipulation(look at Fig.240)

(3)按揉次髎、环跳穴，弹拨臀上皮神经区、臀中肌压痛反应点。

The third Step, the pressing-kneading is given at the points Ciliao and Huantiao, then plucking on the region of the nervi clunium superiors and the trigger points in the gluteus medius.

(4)仰卧，滚腹股沟部至膝上方，上下往返3遍；患肢呈"4"字形，边滚内收肌，边配合压膝扳动(参见图241)。

The fourth step, the patient is in supine position. Rolling is given from groin to superior part of the knee to and fro. for 3 times. With suffered leg put in a shape of "4"mark, then rolling is done on the adductor muscles and coordinated with the wrenching of hip joint as constrained Patrick's test(look at Fig.241).

(5)按揉耻骨梳内收肌压痛反应点。

The fifth step, the pressing-kneading is given on the trigger point of the adductor muscles on the comb of pubis.

(6)侧卧,擦阔筋膜张肌至膝外侧,上下往返3遍,边擦边配合内收髋扳动(图298)。

The sixth step, the patient is in side-lying position. The rolling is done from the tensor fasciae latae to the lateral side of knee up and down for 3 times and coordinated with the adduction-wrenching of the hip(Fig. 298).

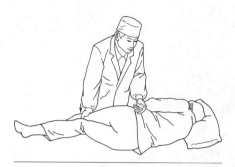

图298 擦股外侧配合内收髋
Fig. 298 Rolling coordinated with adduction — wrenching of hip

(7)按揉阔筋膜张肌压痛反应点。

The seventh step, the pressing-kneading is given at the trigger points along the tensor fasciae latae.

(8)拔伸患肢,根据病理特点,应用骶髂关节、髋关节整复手法(选择性)。

The eighth step, pulling is manipulated on the lower limb and the reduction of the sacroiliac joint or the hip joint is given depended on individual conditions (Selected step).

(9)摇髋关节,抖下肢。

The ninth step, rotating is given on the hip joint, then shaking to finish the routine.

5. 适应证

凡骶髂关节扭伤、臀筋膜劳损、梨状肌综合征、髋关节扭伤、股外侧皮神经炎、内收肌损伤均可以髋臀部常规操作为基本操作程序,并予以增减。

5. Indications

All the sprain of the saroiliac joint, strain of the gluteofascia, pisiform syndrome, sprain of the hip joint, lateral femor cutaneous neuritis and strain of adductor muscles can be treated with this routine, which can be modified, if necessary.

九、膝部操作常规
The Routine Techniques on the Knee Region

1. 体位
卧位。
1. Position
Lying.

2. 重点刺激穴位
健膝、髀关、膝眼、髌骨周缘、委中、委阳。
2. Key points of Stimulation
Jianxi(Extra), Biguan(ST 31), Xiyan(EX–LE 5), Rim of patella, Weizhong(BL 40), Weiyang(BL 39).

3. 主要手法
滚法、按揉、拿法、推扳、环摇。
3. Main manipulations
Rolling, Pressing-kneading, Grasping, Thrusting-wrenching, Rotating.

4. 操作步骤
(1)仰卧。滚股四头肌，自腹股沟至髌骨，上下往返3遍，在髀关、健膝、髌骨内上角处作重点刺激。再按健膝，按揉髌骨周缘，拿起髌骨数次。
4. Manipulation steps
The first step, the patient is in the supine position. The rolling is manipulated on the quadriceps femurs region from the groin to the patella bone to and fro for 3 times. The focal stimulating points are Biguan, Jianxi and the medial superior angle of the patella. Then pressing manipulation is done at the point Jianxi, followed by pressing-kneading on the rim of the patella, grasping on the patella for several times.

(2)滚两膝眼处，配合屈膝扳动(参见图245)。
The second step, rolling is done on the two Xiyan and coordinated with flexion-wrenching of knee(Look at Fig.245).

(3)掌根抵住髌骨下缘向上推，紧张髌韧带，并作快速左右

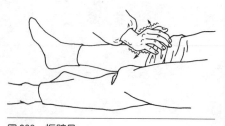

图299 振髌骨
Fig. 299 Vibrating on patella

摆腕振动(图299)。

The third step, the manipulator contacts the lower rim of the patella with palm heel to push it upward to tend the patellar tendon and shakes it rapidly with the movement of swinging wrist(Fig.299).

(4)俯卧,㨰腘绳肌,自坐骨结节至腘窝,上下往返3遍,在委中、委阳处作重点刺激。

The fourth step, the patient lies in the prone position. Rolling is manipulated on the hamstrings region from the tubercle ischia to hollow of the knee to and fro. for 3 to 5 times. The focal stimulating points are Weizhong and Weiyang.

(5)㨰腘窝,配合伸膝扳动(参见图246)。

The fifth step, rolling is done on the hollow of knee and coordinated with the extension wrenching of knee (Look at Fig. 246).

(6)拿大腿,自上而下,从髋关节至膝关节,在重点刺激穴位处停留片刻,加强刺激。

The sixth step, grasping is provided on the thigh from the hip to the knee. As the hand moved at the key points, it is required to halt a moment to strengthen stimulus.

(7)㨰股骨内、外上髁及胫腓骨侧副韧带附着处。

The seventh step, rolling is done at the lateral condyle and the medial condyle of the femur, as well as the lower attaching regions of the collateral ligaments on the tibia and fibula.

(8)屈膝90°,环摇膝关节;搓膝部,擦膝部,抖下肢,结束操作。

The eighth step, kept in 90 degree of flexion, the knee is manipulated with the rotating, then the rubbing with two palms, and then the linear rubbing. Shaking lower limb is done to finish the routine.

5. 适应证

凡膝关节扭伤、膝关节炎、膝关节周围粘连、脂肪垫劳损等病症均可用膝部操作常规作为基本操作法，并适当增减。

5.Indications

All the sprain of the knee joint, knee arthritis, periarthral adhesion of knee, and sprain of the fat-pad can be treated with this routine, which may be modified on the basis of disease character.

十、足踝部操作常规
The Routine Techniques on the Ankle and the Foot Regions

1. 体位

  卧位。

1. Position

  Lying.

2. 重点刺激穴位

  昆仑、太溪、丘墟、照海。

2. Key points of stimulation

  Kunlun (BL 60), Taixi (KI 3), Qiuxu (GB 40) and Zhaohai(KI 6)。

3. 主要手法

  𨰻法、按揉、拿法、拔伸、环摇、推扳、擦法。

3. Main manipulations

  Rolling, Pressing-kneading, Grasping, Pulling, Rotating, Thrusting-wrenching and Linear-rubbing.

4. 操作步骤

  (1) 𨰻胫前肌群至踝关节、足背，上下往返3次；𨰻腓骨肌群至踝关节外侧，上下往返3次；𨰻胫后肌群至踝关节内侧，上下往返3次。

4. Manipulation steps

  The first step, rolling. The rolling is exerted on the region of the anterior muscles of the tibia and the instep to and fro for 3 times, then on the region of the fibular muscles and the lateral side of the foot to and fro for 3 times, and then on the region of posterior muscles of the tibia and the medial side of the foot to and fro for 3 times.

(2)拿小腿，自上而下，在昆仑、太溪、丘墟、照海穴处重点刺激

The second step, grasping is done on the lower leg up-downward. The focal points of stimulating are Kunlun, Taixi, Qiuxu and Zhaohai.

(3)拔伸踝关节，并在拔伸状态下按揉踝关节间隙(图300)

The third Step, pulling is done on the ankle joint for a moment and then followed by pressing-kneading along the articulator interval of the joint while pulling(Fig. 300).

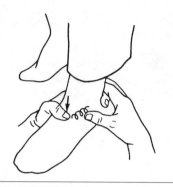

图300 按揉踝关节间隙
Fig. 300 Pressing-kneading along the articulator interval of the joint

(4)滚外踝，配合足内翻扳动(图301)；滚内踝，配合足外翻扳动(图302)；滚跟腱处，配合足背屈扳动(图303)；滚踝关节前方，配合足跖屈扳动(图304)。

The fourth step, rolling is done on the lateral malleolar region and coordinated with supination-wrenching of the foot(Fig.301),on the medial malleolar region with pronation-wrenching of the foot(Fig.302),on the achilles tendon with the extension-wrenching of the ankle(Fig. 303), and last on the anterior region of the ankle with the plantar flexion-wrenching of the ankle (Fig.304).

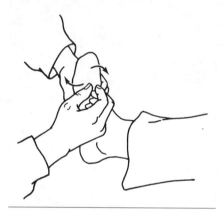

图301 滚外踝配合内翻扳
Fig. 301 Rolling on lateral malleolar coordinated with supination-wrenching

(5)拿揉各跖骨间隙，自近而远；捻各趾。

The fifth step, grasping-kneading is exerted along the intertarsalis spaces proximal to distal. When all the intertarsalis spaces have been stimulated, each toe is manipulated with holding-kneading.

(6)环摇踝关节，擦踝关节间隙，搓踝部，结束治疗。

The sixth step, the ankle joint is ended with the manipulations rotating, linear rubbing and rubbing with two palms.

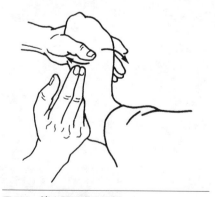

图302 滚内踝配合外翻扳
Fig. 302 Rolling on medial malleolar coordinated with pronation wrenching

5. 适应证

本操作常规适用于踝关节扭伤、踝关节骨关节炎的治疗。也可根据病理特点，予以增减。

5. Indications

This manipulation routine is suitable for the treatments of the sprain of the ankle joint and the ankle osteoarthritis. It should be modified on the basis of pathological characters.

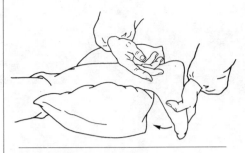

图303 拨跟腱配合伸踝扳
Fig.303 Rolling on achilles tendon coordinated with extension-wrenching

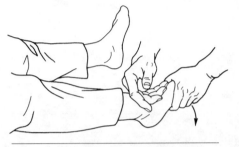

图304 拨踝前方配合跖屈扳
Fig.304 Rolling on instep coordinated with plantar flexion-wrenching